101 Workouts
for Women

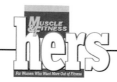

MUSCLE & FITNESS
hers
For Women Who Want More Out of Fitness

101 Workouts
for Women

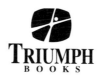

TRIUMPH
BOOKS

By the editors of MUSCLE & FITNESS HERS

Acknowledgments

This publication is based on articles written by Michelle Basta Boubion, NSCA-CPT; Michael Berg, NSCA-CPT; Kira Camp, MS; Allan Donnelly; Tabatha Elliott, PhD; Kathleen Engel; Bill Geiger; Kim Hartt; Lori Incledon, LPTA, CSCS; William Kraemer, PhD, CSCS; Kim Lyons, CPT; Lara McGlashan; Sherri McMillan, CPT; Denise Paglia; Jimmy Peña, MS, CSCS; Linda Shelton; Beth Sonnenburg Saltz, MPH; Steve Stiefel; Melyssa St. Michael, CPT; and Jim Stoppani, PhD.

Cover photography by Jim Purdum.

Photography by Cory Sorensen, Roni Ramos, Per Bernal, Jim Purdum, Ian Logan and Robert Reiff.

Project editors are Kristina Haar and Carey Rossi.

Project design by Michael Touna and Amanda McDermott.

Production manager is Lesley Johnson.

Editor in Chief/Group Editorial Director of MUSCLE & FITNESS HERS is Peter McGough.
Founding Chairman is Joe Weider. President, CEO of American Media, Inc., is David Pecker.

ISBN 978-1-60078-023-3

Printed in the USA.

Contents

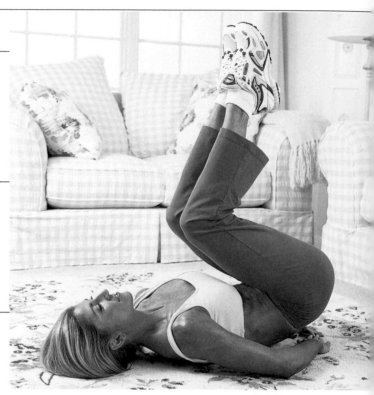

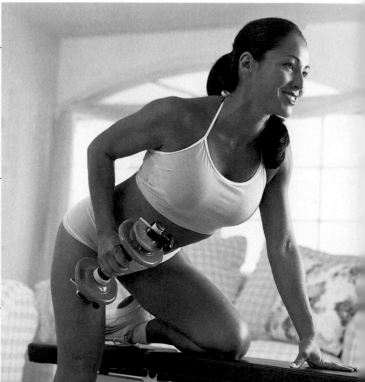

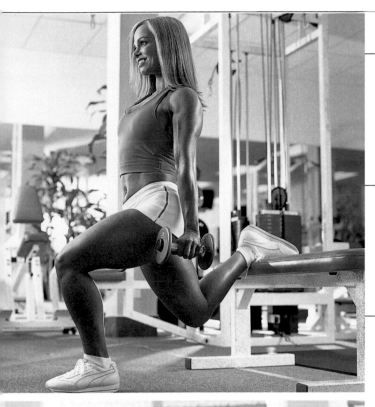

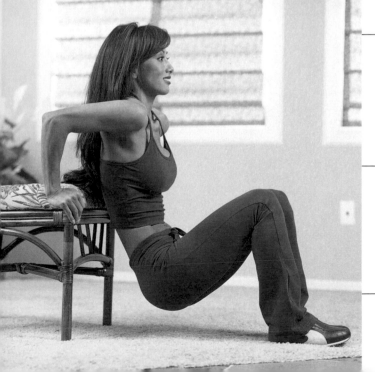

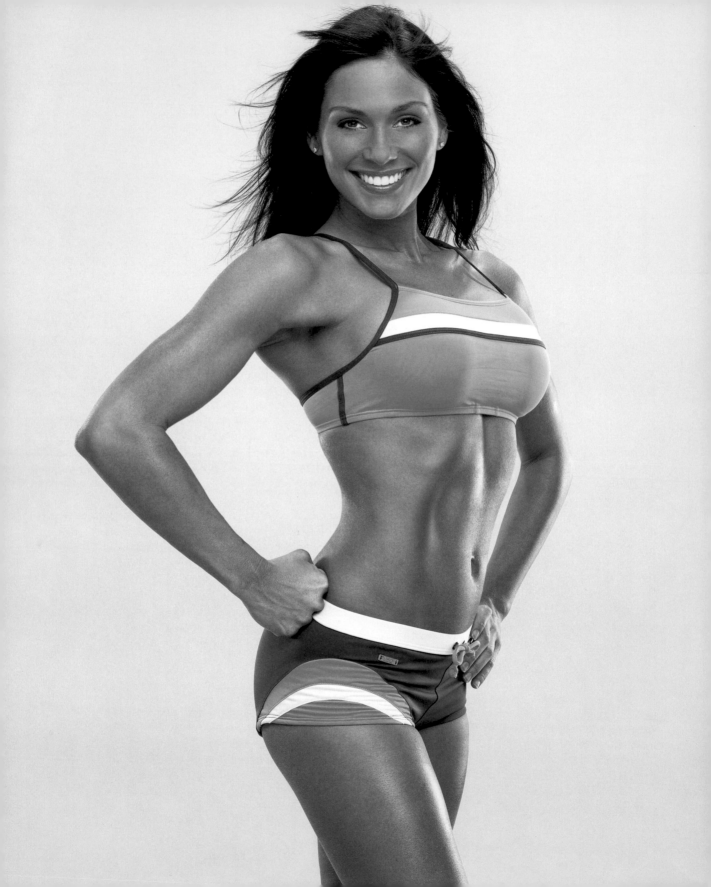

Preface: How to Use This Book

Whether you've just decided to venture into the weight room or you've been making a place for yourself next to the big boys for a while, one thing is certain: You can never have too many workout options.

That's where this book comes in. Here we cut to the chase with 101 different programs delivered straight from the experts at MUSCLE & FITNESS HERS. Whether you want to work your whole body at once or focus on just one bodypart, you'll find a routine for every need and for any day of the week.

You can use this book in a number of different ways. You could:

1 | **Create an all-new bodypart training split based on your goals and your situation.** For instance, if you can only work out at home:
Monday: Chest (p. 78) and Triceps (p. 42)
Tuesday: Legs (p. 142)
Wednesday: Off
Thursday: Back (p. 94) and Biceps (p. 48)
Friday: Shoulders (p. 58) and Abs (p. 12)

2 | **Introduce some variety to your training program, or focus on a particular bodypart that needs attention.** Sometimes, the best way to kick yourself into gear and beat the boredom is to try something new. If you're sick of crunches, turn to the ab chapter and choose one of the 13 workouts

you'll find there, just for today. Or if you aren't developing that cap on your shoulders that helps make your waist and hips look smaller, give them a nudge with the targeted workout on page 68.

3 | **Choose one of the full-body routines,** starting on page 154. Or select an upper-body workout from Chapter 7 and a leg workout from Chapter 6, and do each once or twice per week (for example, Monday and Thursday for upper body, and Tuesday and Friday for the leg workout). Just like that, you've created your own full-body program.

4 | **Perhaps you just want to tweak your workout routine.** In that case, try some new exercises. With nearly 200 illustrated moves in this training manual, you can swap out an exercise or two in your current routine. This is an easy way to introduce variety into your training, in addition to switching up other variables such as sets, reps and exercise order. You'll find plenty of new ideas on all those fronts here.

All told, there are years worth of workouts in this book. We firmly believe it could become the most valuable fitness resource you've ever owned.

The Editors
MUSCLE & FITNESS HERS

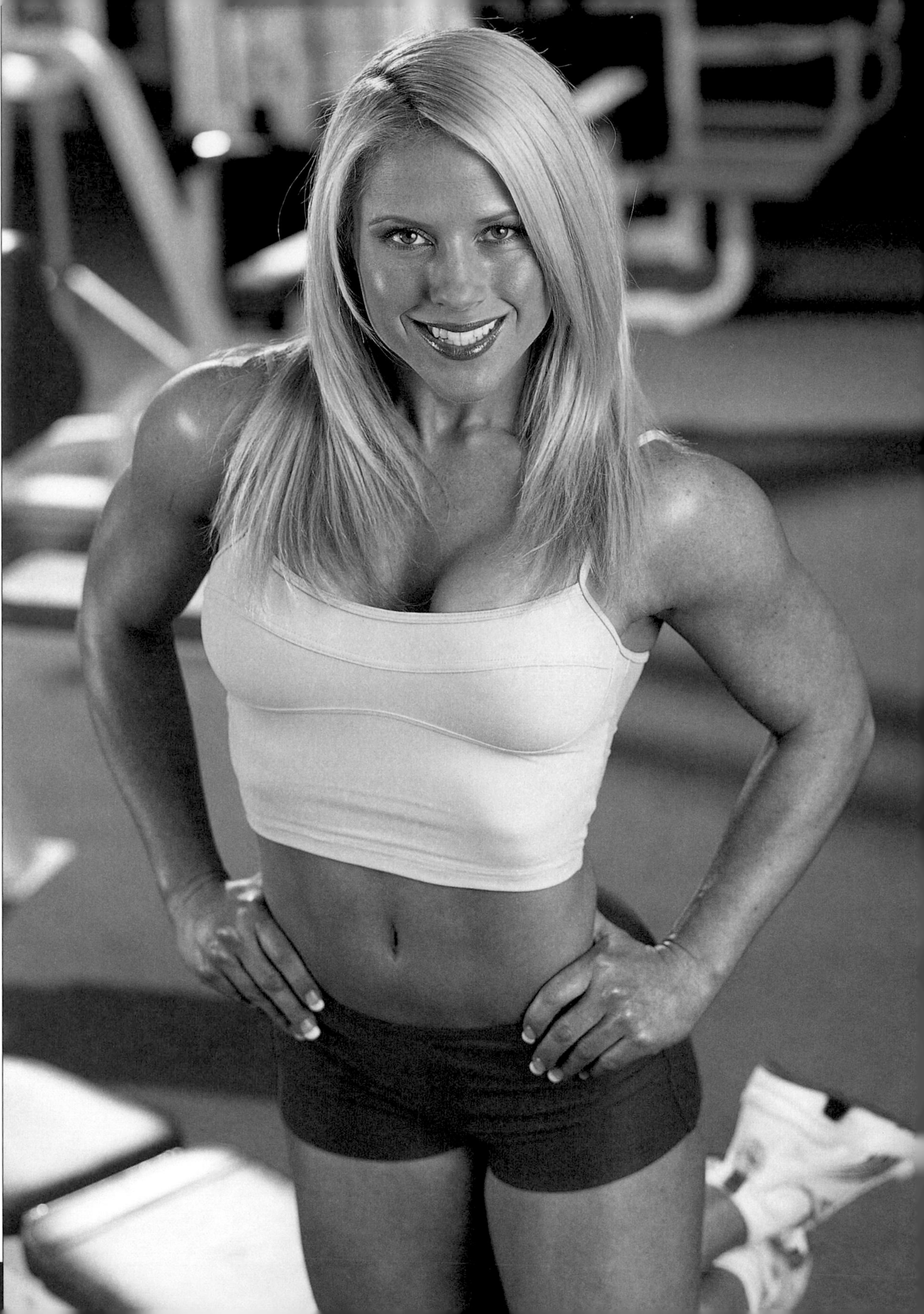

Chapter ONE

Awesome Abdominals

We crave them, we obsess about them and we're constantly holding them in. We're talking about abs, of course. With a solid diet plan and the workouts in this chapter, you too can achieve a head-turning midsection.

GETTING STARTED | Your abs are one of the easiest bodyparts to train at home, and this top-to-bottom routine takes only 15 minutes to complete. Perform each of the exercises 3–4 days a week, periodically swapping out these moves for other favorites.

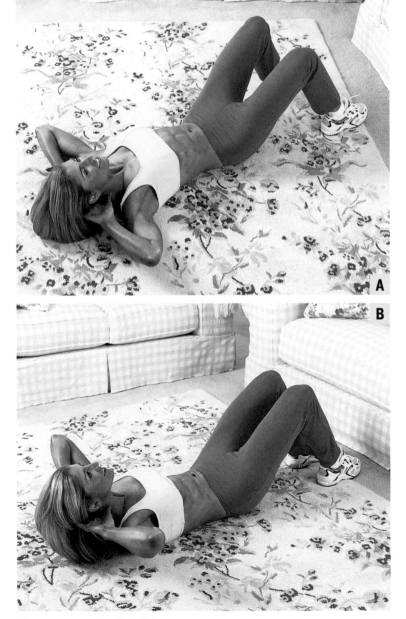

A

B

Crunch

Lie faceup with your knees bent and feet flat on the floor, or bend your knees and bring your feet up in the air. Be sure your lower back is pressed firmly into the floor. Touch your hands behind your head and curl your upper chest toward your hips, lifting your shoulder blades off the floor. For a more advanced move, lift your feet and curl your knees toward your chest as you crunch your torso up. Squeeze your abs before lowering back to the start.

Double Crunch

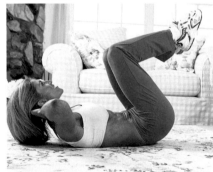

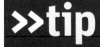

As you become more advanced, increase the reps to 20–25. Correct technique should bring you to muscle failure. If you feel you can do more, you may need to tighten your form.

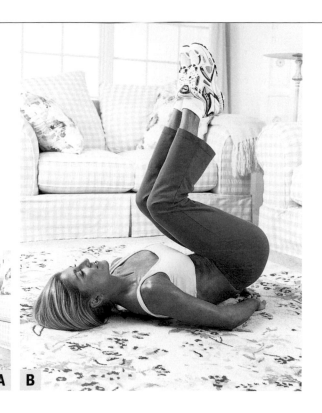

A **B**

Reverse Crunch

Begin by lying faceup on the floor. Bend your knees, lift your legs 90 degrees from your hips and place your hands under your lower back. Contract through your lower abs to slowly curl your pelvis off the floor and toward your ribcage, holding for a moment at the top. Slowly lower your legs and hips back to the start position.

Side-to-Side Crunch

Start in the same position as the crunch. Support your head by placing your hands lightly behind it, then lift your head and shoulder blades off the floor. Hold this position and crunch to your right side to work your obliques, thinking of bringing your right elbow to your right hip while keeping your lower back pressed firmly against the floor. Repeat to the left side. Your abs will perform an isometric contraction as you hold your head and shoulder blades off the floor, putting the muscular stress on the obliques.

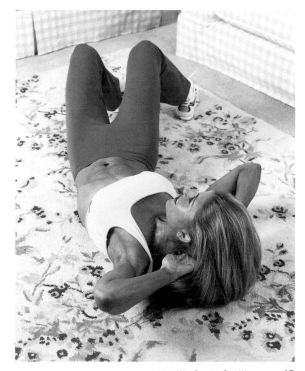

At-Home Ab/Oblique Routine

Exercise	Sets	Reps
Crunch	3	10–15
Reverse Crunch	3	10–15
Side-to-Side Crunch	3	10–15*
*each side		

GETTING STARTED | Get your heart rate up and melt the flab that's covering your abs with this routine. Perform the exercises one right after the other, moving quickly from one to the next. This continuous movement will keep your body warm and working hard.

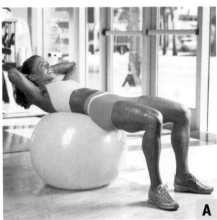 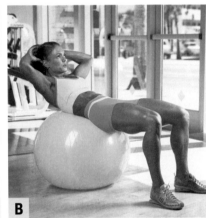

A **B**

Exercise-Ball Crunch

Lie back on an exercise ball so your torso is parallel to the floor, feet hip-width apart and knees bent 90 degrees. Press your lower back into the ball and place your hands lightly behind your head. Lift your shoulders while keeping your hips stationary. Squeeze your abs briefly at the top, then slowly return to the start position and repeat without bouncing or pausing. Be sure you crunch by flexing your spine, not your hips.

Exercise-Ball Oblique Crunch

Lie back on an exercise ball, torso parallel to the floor, hands lightly behind your head. Lift your shoulders by contracting your abs, then twist your torso to aim your left shoulder toward your right knee. Hold briefly, return to the neutral crunched position, then slowly return to the start position. Alternate reps to each side.

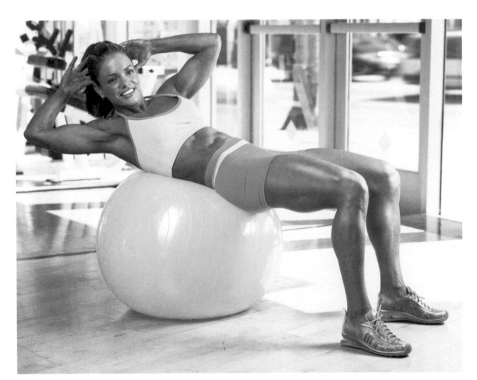

Cable Crunch

Attach either a close-grip handle or a rope to a high-pulley cable. Facing the weight stack, step back 2–3 feet and kneel down, taking a firm grip with both hands in front of you and leaning forward slightly. Keep your lower body stationary as you contract your abs and aim your elbows toward your knees to curl your torso toward the floor. Squeeze your abs briefly, then slowly return to the start position.

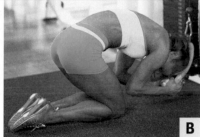

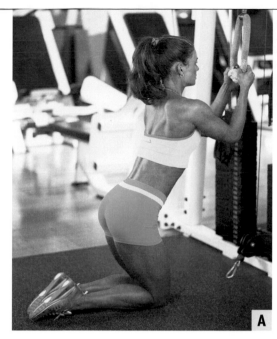

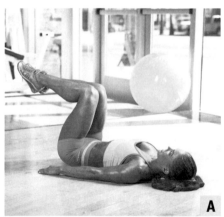

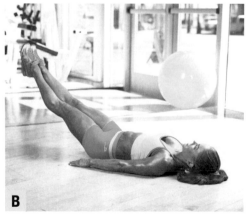

Kick-Out

Lie faceup on the floor with your knees and hips bent 90 degrees. Place your hands down by your sides and extend your legs straight out at about a 45-degree angle. Hold this position for a count, then slowly return to the start. Repeat for reps without letting your feet touch the floor.

Giant-Set Ab Routine

Exercise	Sets	Reps
Exercise-Ball Crunch	3	20–25
Exercise-Ball Oblique Crunch	3	20–25*
Cable Crunch	3	20–25
Kick-Out	3	20–25

Quickly move from exercise to exercise, resting no more than 30 seconds between a set for each one. Do the entire circuit three times. You can rest between circuits, but only for a minute or two.
*each side

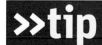

>>tip

Exercise balls come in a variety of sizes, but as a general rule of thumb, when you sit on a ball, your knees should be even with or slightly below your hips.

GETTING STARTED | Most of us know exactly when we last did crunches, but when was the last time you worked your lower back? Training one but not the other leads to an imbalance, which you may not even recognize because your body adapts to these changes over time.

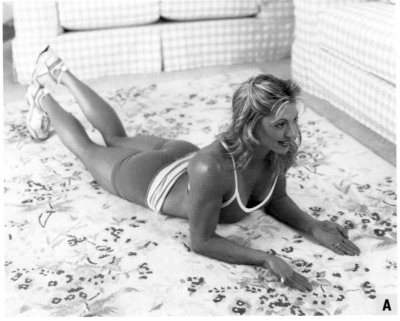

A

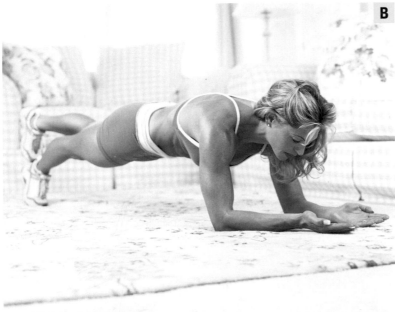

B

Combination Stabilizer

Lie facedown on the floor, resting on your elbows with your arms tight by your sides and palms facing up. Place your left toes on top of your right heel. Using your abdominal and back muscles, push through your hips to lift your torso off the floor. Hold this position for as long as you can (at least a minute) before returning to the start. Switch foot position and repeat.

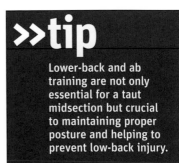

>>tip

Lower-back and ab training are not only essential for a taut midsection but crucial to maintaining proper posture and helping to prevent low-back injury.

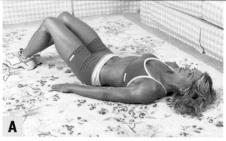

Bent-Knee V-Up

Lie faceup with your arms down by your sides, knees bent and feet on the floor. Simultaneously lift your knees toward your chest and crunch your upper body forward. Lower back to the start, keeping your heels and shoulder blades off the floor. Focus your eyes above your knees to keep your chin off your chest.

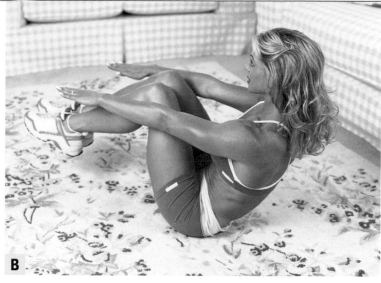

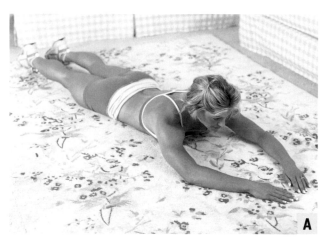

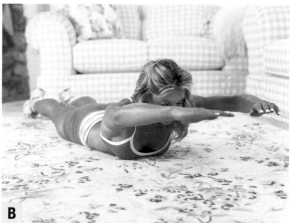

Superman

Lie facedown on the floor with your arms extended out in front, elbows slightly bent. Using your lower-back muscles, lift your chest off the floor, keeping your neck and arms in line with your spine. Avoid lifting your legs and chest simultaneously; this can put too much pressure on the discs in your back.

At-Home Ab/Low-Back Routine

Exercise	Sets	Reps
Combination Stabilizer	3	1 minute*
Bent-Knee V-Up	3	10
Superman	3	1 minute
*each side		

GETTING STARTED | With ab training, it's the negative that counts — the negative or eccentric contraction, that is. Perform each movement in two parts, holding the top position for one count and moving slowly through the negative rep to return to the start in two counts.

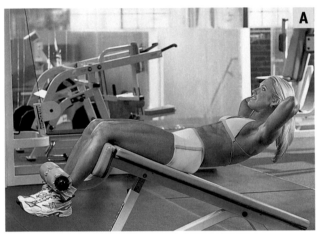

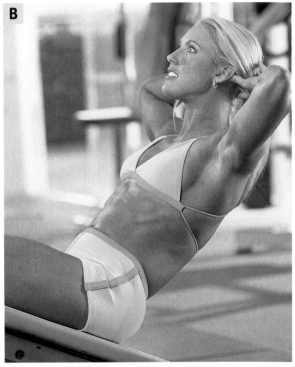

Decline-Bench Crunch

Sit upright on the bench with your feet under the rollers, keeping your feet and lower legs relaxed. Place your hands lightly behind your head, which increases the resistance against which your abs will move. Lower yourself slowly and under control, holding your abs tight throughout. Think about making your torso as long as possible throughout the negative rep. At the bottom, keep your abs tight as you begin to shift direction. Curl up until you're just short of vertical, using the strength of your abs rather than leverage against the footpad.

>>tip

Instead of relaxing your muscles on the return, really focus on and emphasize the negative phase of the rep. It's an oft-overlooked but particularly important aspect of sculpting great abs.

Hip Thrust

Lie faceup on a flat bench, grasping its edges alongside your head. Start with your legs straight and elevated at about a 90-degree angle. Using a moderate pace, contract your abs to raise your hips off the bench about 2–3 inches. Lower slowly and go straight into the next rep.

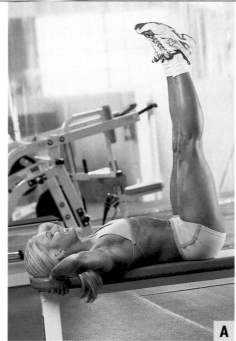
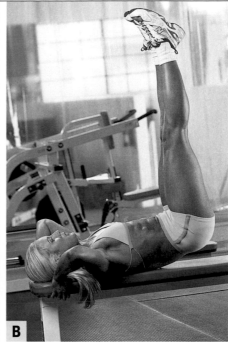

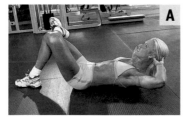
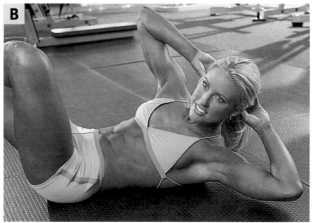

Cross-Body Crunch

Lie faceup on the floor, cross one foot over the opposite knee and place both hands lightly behind your head. Curl up using the strength of your abs to lift your shoulder blades off the floor, then twist your torso to bring one shoulder as far as possible toward the opposite knee. Lower slowly, keeping your abs tight on the return. Alternate reps to each side.

Ab & Oblique Routine

Exercise	Sets	Reps
Cross-Body Crunch	2	15*
Decline-Bench Crunch	3	8–10
Hip Thrust	3	10
*each side		

GETTING STARTED | The exercise ball or stability ball is a great tool for training abs. Performing these common core exercises on a ball recruits and fatigues more muscle fibers to help you keep your balance, with the added benefit of firming your entire midsection.

Exercise-Ball Back Extension

Stand facing away from a wall in front of an exercise ball. Lie facedown over the ball so your midsection is fully supported. With your feet against the wall, hands lightly behind your head and abs tight throughout, slowly raise your torso to a comfortable position before returning to the start.

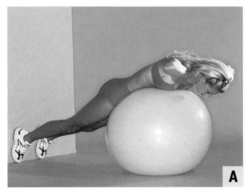

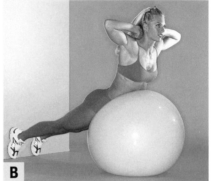

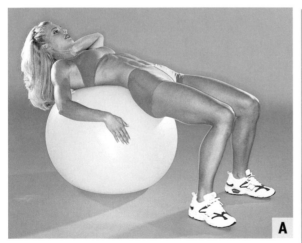

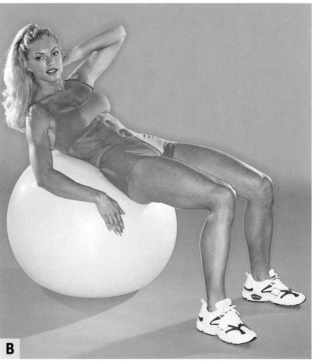

Exercise-Ball Oblique Crunch

Lie faceup over an exercise ball, finding a position in which the ball comfortably supports your low back. Tuck your chin in slightly, focusing your eyes at a 45-degree angle — roughly the point at which ceiling meets wall. Keeping your abs contracted throughout, slowly crunch your ribcage in a diagonal direction, moving one shoulder toward the opposite hip. Repeat for reps, then switch sides.

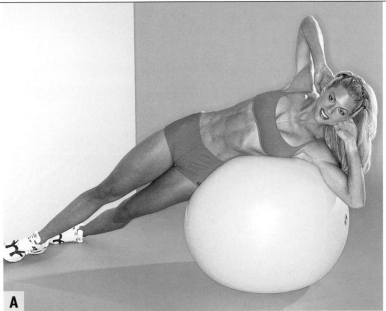

A

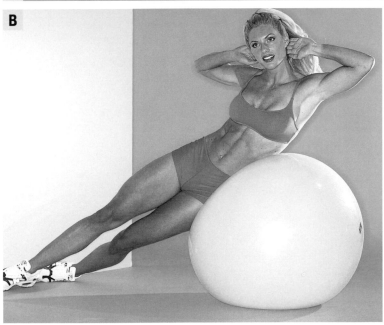

B

Exercise-Ball Lateral Abdominal Flexion

Lie sideways over an exercise ball with your legs extended out to the side, feet against the wall. Keeping your abs contracted and your hands lightly behind your head, slowly crunch up sideways, making sure not to simultaneously flex your torso forward or backward. Repeat for reps, then switch sides.

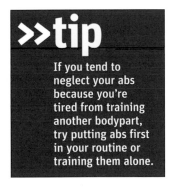

>>tip

If you tend to neglect your abs because you're tired from training another bodypart, try putting abs first in your routine or training them alone.

Exercise-Ball Ab Routine

Exercise	Sets	Reps
Exercise-Ball Crunch	3	8–15
Exercise-Ball Oblique Crunch	3	8–15*
Exercise-Ball Back Extension	3	8–15
Exercise-Ball Lateral Abdominal Flexion	3	8–15*

*each side

GETTING STARTED | When it comes to getting a drum-tight midsection, it's important to work both the six-pack muscles — the upper and lower abs and the oblique muscles along each side. This workout does just that with exercises that target each region.

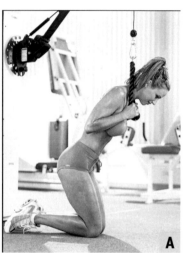

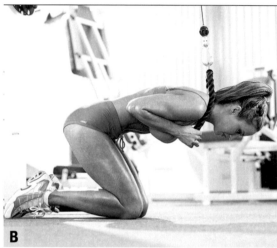

Cable Crunch

Kneel facing a cable station with a rope handle attached to the upper-pulley cable. Place the rope behind your head and hold the ends near your collarbones; lean forward slightly. Crunch down, aiming your forehead toward the floor while keeping your lower body and arms stationary.

Straight-Leg Crunch

Lie faceup on the floor with your legs straight up in the air, perpendicular to your torso. Extend your arms toward your feet and reach for your toes as you crunch up to raise your shoulders off the floor. Contract your abs tighter at the top, then reverse the motion, but don't go all the way back down.

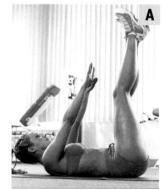

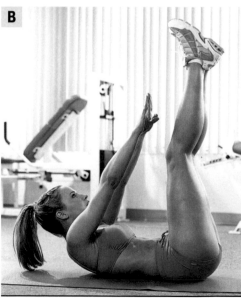

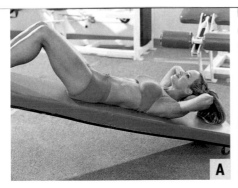
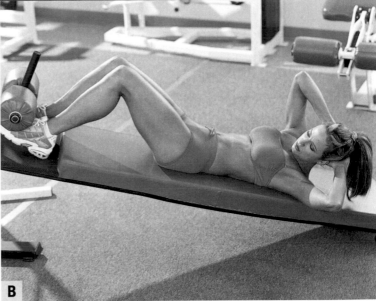

Decline Twist Crunch

Set a decline bench to 30–35 degrees and secure your feet under the rollers. With your knees bent 90 degrees and your hands lightly supporting your head, lie back slowly. Crunch back up, aiming your right shoulder toward your left hip. Complete all reps for one side, then switch sides.

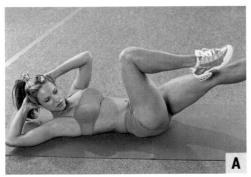
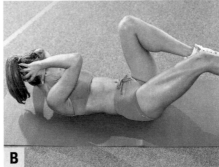

Bicycle

Lie faceup on the floor with your knees bent, feet up off the floor and hands lightly behind your head. Crunch up and aim your left shoulder toward your right knee while pulling that knee in. Alternate from side to side, keeping the motion smooth and controlled.

>>tip

Challenge your ab muscles by keeping your shoulder blades off the floor and the weight plates off the stack between reps. Switch the order of exercises each time you do your workout.

Ab & Oblique Routine

Exercise	Sets	Reps
Cable Crunch	3	15–20
Straight-Leg Crunch	3	15–20
Decline Twist Crunch	3	15–20*
Bicycle	3	15–20*

*each side

GETTING STARTED | If you've worked to whittle your middle but have little muscle to show for it, the time has come. This routine will overload your ab muscles using high reps. Paired with a lean diet and cardio, you can turn your tummy into a trophy of dedication.

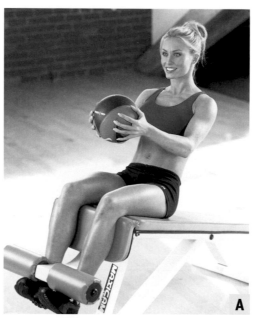

Decline Weighted Twist

This exercise will stimulate your entire core. Grasp a weight plate or a medicine ball and sit upright on a decline bench, feet secured. Lean back until your torso is perpendicular to the bench (A). Holding the weight/ball out in front of your body, gently twist to the right (B) and then to the left (C). This exercise is great for the oblique muscles, which don't follow a straight line between origin and insertion but instead wrap around the torso.

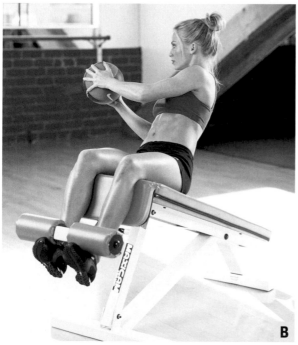

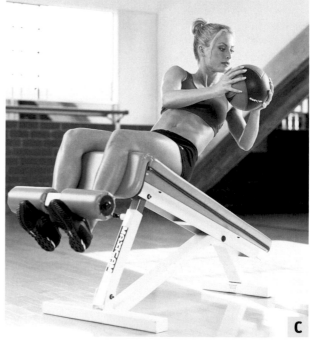

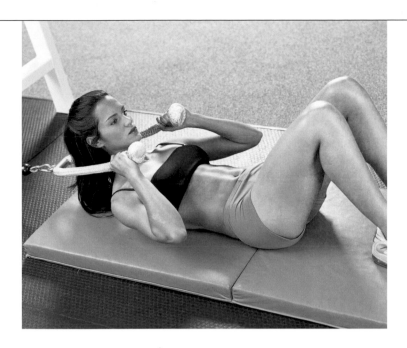

Lying Cable Crunch

Lie faceup on the floor with your head roughly a foot in front of and facing away from the weight stack of a cable station, knees bent and feet flat on the floor. Grasp the rope attached to the low-pulley cable and bring your hands above your collarbones; your head will be inside the V of the rope. Perform a standard crunch, bringing your head and shoulders off the floor. Squeeze at the top of the movement and slowly return to the start. Try not to let the weight touch the stack, and keep your hands close to your body throughout the set.

Scissor-to-a-Crunch

Lie faceup on the floor with your legs straight, heels about 6 inches off the floor (A). Separate your legs as far apart as possible (B) and then bring them back together, but don't cross them. With your feet together, bend your knees and bring them into your chest while crunching up with your upper body (C). In sequence: heels up, legs apart, legs together, double crunch, then repeat. Try not to let your heels or legs touch the floor.

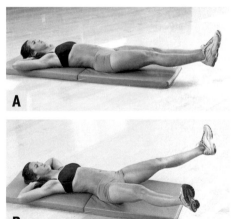

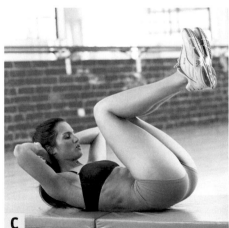

High-Rep Ab/Oblique Routine

Exercise	Sets	Reps
Decline Weighted Twist	3–4	25
Scissor-to-a-Crunch	3–4	25–30
Lying Cable Crunch	3	25–30

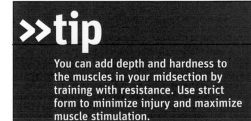

>>tip

You can add depth and hardness to the muscles in your midsection by training with resistance. Use strict form to minimize injury and maximize muscle stimulation.

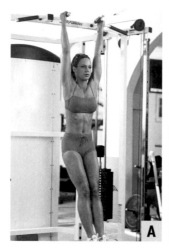

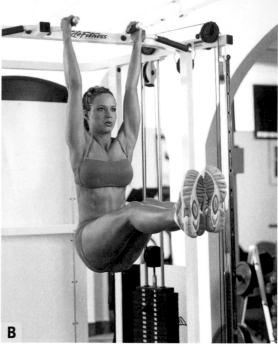

GETTING STARTED | If you have the exercises from Workout 6 down pat, it's time to kick it up a notch by building on that base. The basic crunch is made more difficult by straightening your arms overhead, and the cable crunch is modified to target the obliques.

Hanging Leg Raise

Hang from a pull-up bar with your arms and legs fully extended. Without using momentum, contract your abs and raise your legs straight out in front of you till they're parallel to the floor. Return to the start position slowly and under control. Avoid swinging.

A **B**

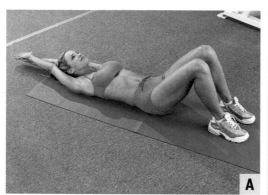

A

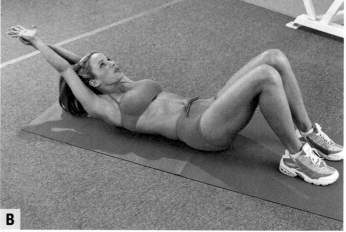

B

Hands-Overhead Crunch

Lie faceup on the floor with your knees bent and feet flat on the floor. Raise your hands overhead and lay one hand on top of the other. Keeping your arms extended, crunch up, lifting your shoulders off the floor. Squeeze your abs at the top, then lower slowly without going all the way down.

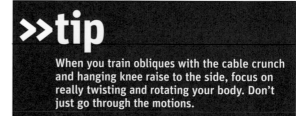

>>tip

When you train obliques with the cable crunch and hanging knee raise to the side, focus on really twisting and rotating your body. Don't just go through the motions.

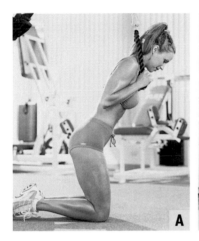

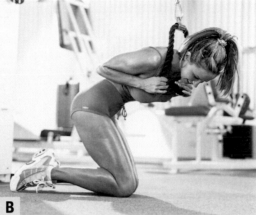

Cable Crossover Crunch

Kneel facing a cable station with a rope handle attached to the upper-pulley cable. Hold the ends near your collarbones and lean slightly forward. Crunch down against the resistance, aiming your left shoulder toward your right hip while keeping your lower body stationary. Alternate reps from side to side.

Hanging Knee Raise to the Side

Hang from a pull-up bar with your arms and legs fully extended. Without using momentum, contract your abs and obliques and raise your knees to your right side as high as you can. Return to the start position slowly and under control, and alternate reps from side to side.

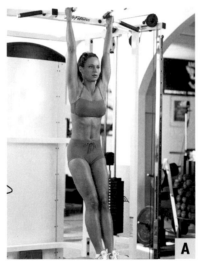

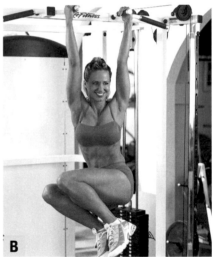

Intermediate Ab & Oblique Routine

Exercise	Sets	Reps
Hands-Overhead Crunch	3	15
Hanging Leg Raise	3	15
Hanging Knee Raise to Side	3	15*
Cable Crossover Crunch	3	15*

*each side

GETTING STARTED | The exercises in this routine target the stabilizing muscles in your low back and abs, conditioning your midsection while reducing your risk of developing back pain. Not only will you strengthen your core but you'll also stand a bit taller.

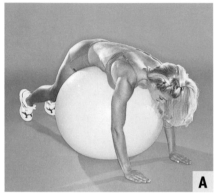 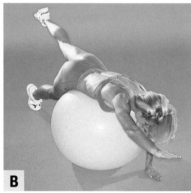

Exercise-Ball Opposite Arm/Leg Lift

Lie facedown on an exercise ball so your midsection is fully supported. Place your hands on the floor underneath your shoulders; position your feet so they also touch the floor. Keep your abs contracted. Without moving your back and keeping your neck neutral, slowly lift one arm and the opposite leg simultaneously. Think about lengthening those limbs rather than lifting them as high as you can. Repeat for reps, then switch sides.

Exercise-Ball Trunk Slide

Kneel down facing an exercise ball and place your clasped hands atop it. Keeping your abs contracted and your back flat, slowly roll the ball forward so that your body moves forward with it. Roll as far as you can without feeling shoulder discomfort or pulling your spine out of position.

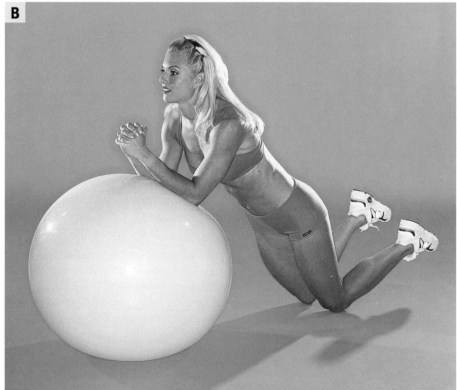

Exercise-Ball Plank-to-Knee Tuck

To start, lie facedown on an exercise ball so your midsection is fully supported. Place your palms flat on the floor — arms straight but not locked — and extend your legs behind you. Using your hands, slowly "walk" yourself forward until your shins rest atop the ball. Keep your hands aligned under your shoulders, your shoulder blades pulled back and your abs contracted. Practice holding this "plank" position for 30–60 seconds, breathing comfortably. For a greater challenge, start in the "plank" position. Draw your knees toward your chest, allowing the ball to roll forward under your shins. Slowly extend your legs back to the start position, keeping your abs contracted and your back flat throughout.

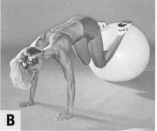

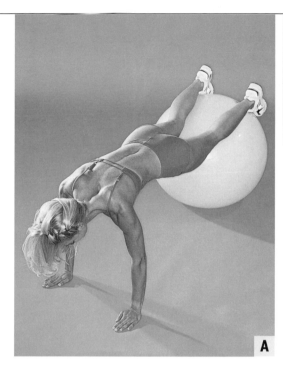

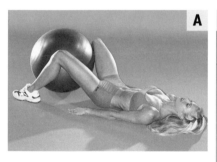

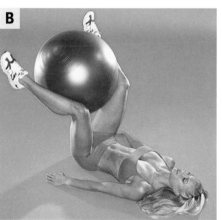

Exercise-Ball Leg Lift

Lie faceup with your feet on the floor, knees bent and an exercise ball positioned between your knees and lower legs. Keeping your abs contracted, slowly lift your feet and the ball off the floor till your thighs are perpendicular. Resist the tendency to arch your back and let your abs protrude. Keep your neck relaxed and your head in contact with the floor. To intensify this movement, lift your feet only a few inches.

>>tip

Before embarking on this program, practice sitting on the ball and getting into the exercises' start positions until you're comfortable keeping your balance.

Exercise-Ball Ab Routine

Exercise	Sets	Reps
Exercise-Ball Opposite Arm/Leg Lift	3	10*
Exercise-Ball Trunk Slide	3	8–12
Exercise-Ball Plank-to-Knee Tuck	3	8–12
Exercise-Ball Leg Lift	3	8–15

Rest 30 seconds between each exercise.
*each side

GETTING STARTED | Bored with traditional ab routines and exercises? Spice up your mid-section training by grabbing a medicine ball and enlisting the help of a friend. Your core development will benefit from these variations as your gym time becomes more fun!

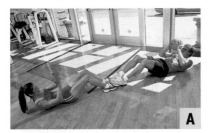

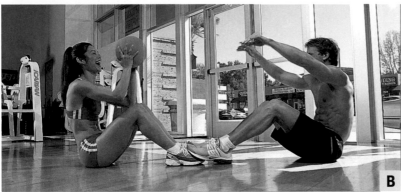

Medicine-Ball Sit-Up/Throw

Both you and your partner lie faceup with your knees bent 90 degrees, feet on the floor, keeping your low backs in contact with the floor. Place your feet atop your partner's or vice versa. You hold the ball. Simultaneously crunch up slowly, lifting one vertebra at a time off the floor. At about 30 degrees you'll reach a sticking point where it feels as though you can't rise any higher. Try to keep going, as high as you can, but don't bounce, use momentum or lift your feet. At the top, throw the ball in chest-press fashion to your partner, who catches it before you both slowly return to the start position. Repeat the ascent so your partner can throw the ball back to you. Take 4–5 seconds each on the way up and down, moving in a controlled manner. Repeat the sequence for reps.

Medicine-Ball Crunch/Leg Lift

Both you and your partner lie faceup with your knees bent 90 degrees, feet on the floor so they almost touch. Start by holding the medicine ball between your feet. Both of you slowly crunch up to a comfortable position while lifting your feet and the ball a few inches; the angle in your knees should stay the same. Slowly return to the start and drop the ball, allowing your partner to pick it up with his/her feet. Repeat the sequence for reps.

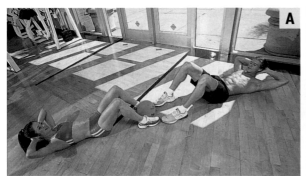

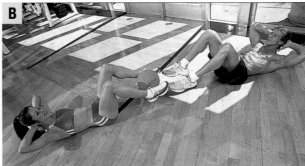

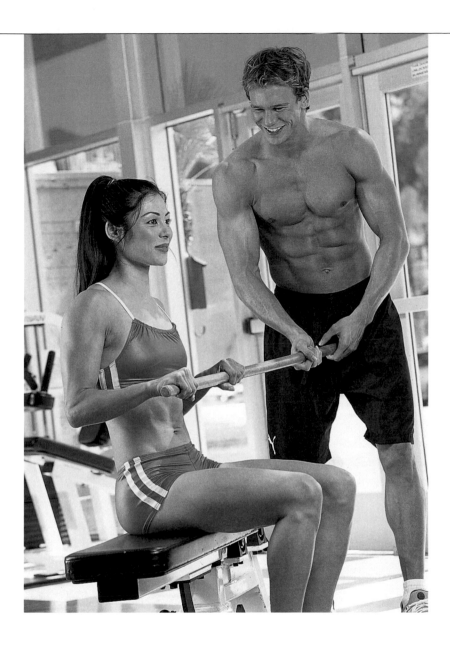

Pole Play

Start by sitting erect on a flat bench with perfect posture and your abs contracted. Firmly hold a broomstick with both hands below your chest and close to your body. Your partner stands to the side and grasps the other end of the stick. The object of the exercise is for your partner to try to move you by pulling and pushing the stick while you try to stay completely stable. Your partner should change the angle of pull regularly to keep you working.

>>tip

Training with a friend can help motivate you and push you to intensity levels that you may not work at on your own.

Partnered Ab Routine

Exercise	Sets	Reps
Medicine-Ball Sit-Up/Throw	2–3	8–15
Medicine-Ball Crunch/Leg Lift	2–3	8–15
Pole Play	2–3	90 sec.*
*per person		

GETTING STARTED | Unfortunately, you need more than the trusty crunch to sculpt awesome abs. You need to literally "go deep" to the internal obliques and transverse abdominis with stabilization exercises such as these. Get ready to work your abs from the inside out.

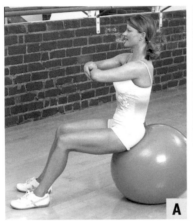
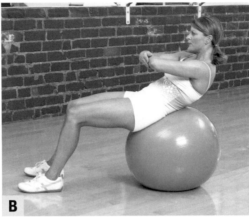

A B

Half Roll-Back on Exercise Ball

Sit upright on the ball as if you were sitting on the edge of a chair, with your feet in front of you for stability and a bit wider than hip-width apart. Roll your glutes up and under you, tilting your pelvis. You should feel the ball rolling under your low back. Try to press one vertebra at a time into the ball. Squeeze your abs as you come back up to the start position.

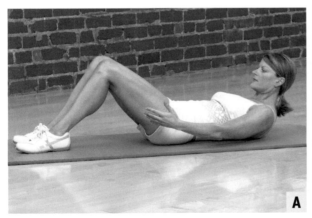
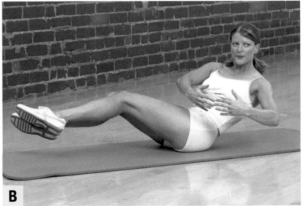

A B

The Sidewinder

Lie faceup on the floor with your knees bent, arms down by your sides, feet flat on the mat and shoulders just off the floor. Crunch up slightly as you lift your feet, squeezing your knees together. Rotate onto your right hip and twist your torso in the opposite direction. Try to keep your abs as tight as possible. When you rotate and get up on your hip, hold for a count of one-one-thousand. If this is too difficult, bend your knees. Come back to the start and alternate sides, returning to the start after each rep.

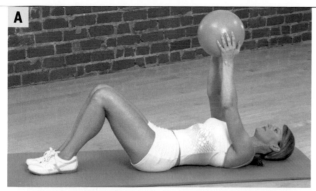

A

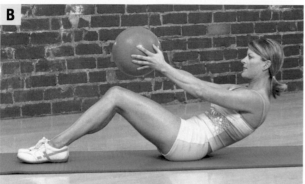

B

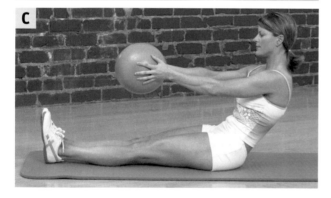

C

The Coil

You should have a feeling of reaching and lengthening during this movement. It's a slow exercise, taking about four seconds up and four seconds down. The return is the most important part of the move as you engage your muscles to resist gravity.

Lying faceup on the floor, begin with your knees bent and feet flat on the mat. Hold a medicine ball above your chest, arms extended (A). Raise your shoulders off the floor and begin to coil up, pushing your low back firmly into the mat (B). To ensure good form, pretend there's a big ball on your midsection and you're trying to go up and over the ball. When the medicine ball nears your knees, begin to slowly straighten your legs. Reach all the way over until the ball nears your toes, keeping your legs straight (C). On the return, bow out your back and scoot your pelvis under you. Try to put one vertebra down at a time. When your middle back reaches the floor, quickly bend your knees and drag your feet toward your glutes.

Deep-Muscle Giant-Set Ab Routine

Perform these three movements in a giant set — a series of exercises done consecutively — in the following order:

Exercise	Sets	Reps
Half Roll-Back on Exercise Ball	2	10
The Sidewinder	2	10
The Coil	2	10*

You may have to work up to this rep range, especially with the more difficult movements. Each exercise should flow into the next, with little rest in between. Each giant set should take 5–6 minutes. Perform each movement slowly and deliberately.
*Rest 30 seconds after the first five reps.

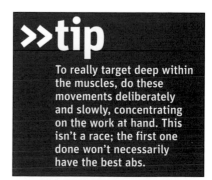

>>tip

To really target deep within the muscles, do these movements deliberately and slowly, concentrating on the work at hand. This isn't a race; the first one done won't necessarily have the best abs.

GETTING STARTED | By now you should feel right at home on the exercise ball. Balance is key for these first two movements as you work to strengthen your core, and your coordination and muscle endurance will be tested with the final two exercises. Get ready to feel the burn.

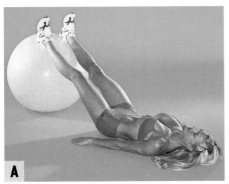

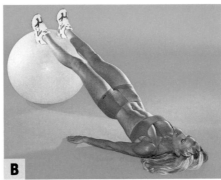

Exercise-Ball Lying Bridge

Lie faceup on the floor with your feet atop an exercise ball and your arms down by your sides. Slowly raise your hips toward the ceiling while contracting your glutes and hamstrings until your bodyweight rests comfortably on your shoulder blades. Return slowly to the start position. Keep your hips square to the ceiling and your abs contracted.

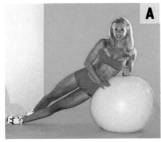

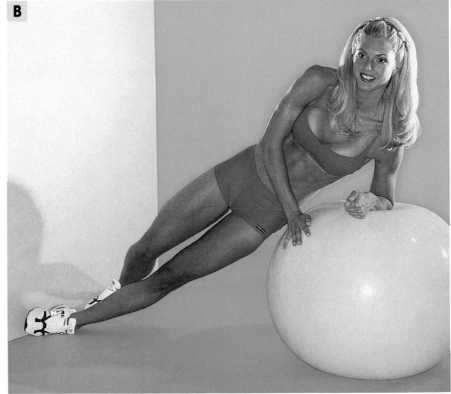

Exercise-Ball Side-Lying Stabilization

Lie on one side over an exercise ball with your legs straight and your feet against a wall. Prop yourself up on one elbow with your hip and side touching the ball. Slowly lift your hip off the ball so that your body is now supported on your elbow and feet, and hold for five seconds. (You can place your free hand on the ball for balance, not leverage.) Keep your abs contracted throughout the exercise. Repeat for reps, then switch sides.

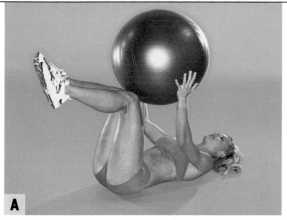

A

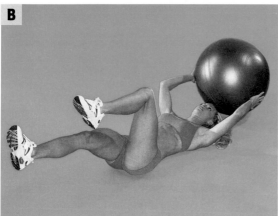

B

Exercise-Ball
Alternating Leg Extension

Lie faceup on the floor holding an exercise ball at arm's length over your abs. Lift your legs and bend your knees so that your knees and hips form 90-degree angles. Tighten your abs and brace your spine. Slowly extend one leg to a 45-degree angle while simultaneously lowering the ball overhead toward the floor. Return to the start position and switch legs. That's one rep.

Exercise-Ball
Rotational V-Sits

Sit upright on the floor holding the exercise ball in front of you, knees bent slightly and heels on the floor. With your bodyweight supported on your glutes, chest out, shoulders back and abs contracted, recline back a few inches. Hold this position as you slowly rotate the ball from side to side, touching the floor with it if you can. Both sides is one rep.

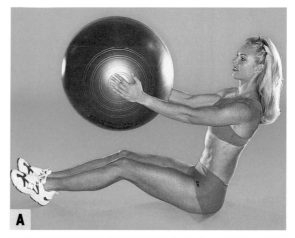

A

B

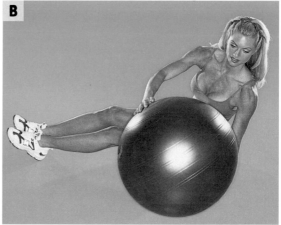

Exercise-Ball Ab Routine

Exercise	Sets	Reps
Exercise-Ball Lying Bridge	3	13–20
Exercise-Ball Side-Lying Stabilization	3	8*
Exercise-Ball Alternating Leg Extension	3	8–15
Exercise-Ball Rotational V-Sits	3	8–15

Rest 30 seconds between each exercise.
*each side

GETTING STARTED | Here's the toughest workout in our bag of flat-ab tricks, and the results are gut-wrenching. Use this routine after you've been training for at least six months to shock your midsection into six-pack shape. Start with one set of each exercise.

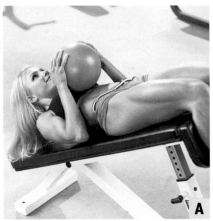
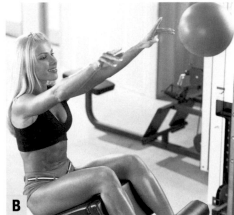

Decline Ball Toss

Lie faceup on a decline bench while your partner stands near your feet with a medicine ball. Sit up to catch the ball your partner tosses you, bring the ball to your chest, roll all the way down and then back up. On the way up, toss the ball to your partner, who catches it and throws it right back. To make it easier, keep the ball at your chest.

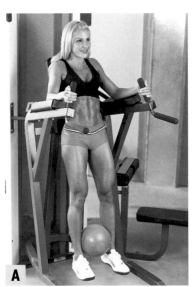
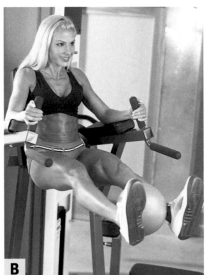
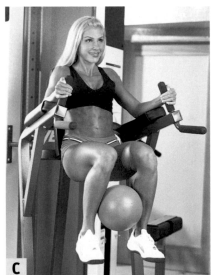

Weighted Leg Raise/Knee-Up Combo

Get into position on the vertical bench, squeezing a medicine ball between your ankles (A). Lift your legs straight up until they're parallel to the floor (B). Once in this L-position, bend your knees and pause (C) before curling your knees up to your chest, pulling in your pelvis and rolling your hips under while squeezing your lower abs (not shown). Make sure your upper back stays flat against the bench throughout the exercise.

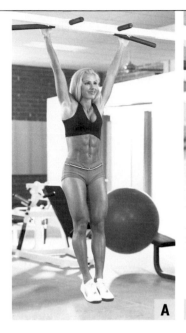
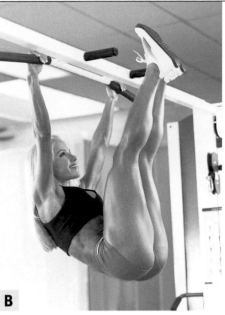

A **B**

Hanging Straight-Leg Raise

Hang from a pull-up bar with your feet off the floor. Try to lift your feet all the way up to the bar before lowering them back down, keeping your legs straight the entire time. Avoid using momentum. To make it more difficult, go superslow. If you tend to lose your grip before your abs fatigue, use straps.

Extreme Decline Crunch

Sit upright on a decline bench with your feet secured under the rollers. Hold a medicine ball on your lap, then crunch your abs so you're hunched over. Keeping your abs contracted, lean back slightly while raising the ball overhead. Gradually straighten your torso so that your back is flat and perpendicular to the bench. Then reverse the extension, curling your torso and crunching toward your hips while bringing the medicine ball back to the start position.

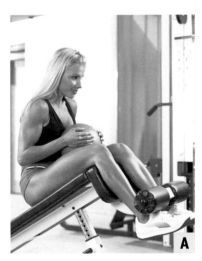
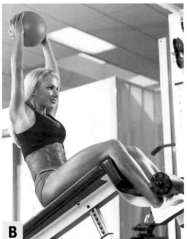

A **B**

Advanced Ab Routine

Exercise	Sets	Reps
Weighted Leg Raise/ Knee-Up Combo	3	20
Decline Ball Toss	4–6	15–20
Hanging Straight-Leg Raise	3	15–20
Extreme Decline Crunch	4	20–30

>>tip

These moves are extremely difficult. If you've never done them before, try doing one set of one exercise at a time without weight on days you train legs, and work your way up.

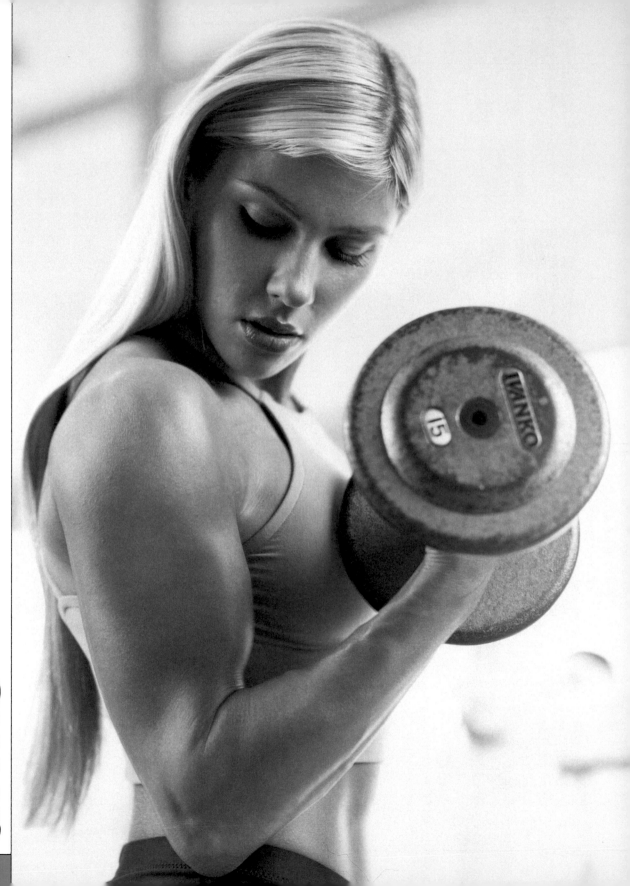

arms

Chapter TWO

Biceps & Triceps

From sports enthusiast to soccer mom, tight, toned arms are a badge of honor. Since everyday activities provide some resistance, sculpting all the right areas means targeted workouts that keep your bi's and tri's long, lean and strong.

GETTING STARTED | When it comes to training biceps, the ability to gain strength comes down to a solid workout plan that varies the equipment and angles used. Start by alternating between these two routines to isolate and shape this coveted arm muscle.

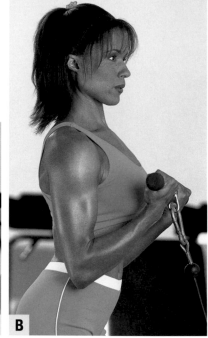

Standing Cable Curl

Stand erect facing a cable station with a short bar attached to the low-pulley cable. With your abs pulled in and shoulders back, lock your elbows by your sides. Contract your biceps and bend your elbows to curl the bar toward your shoulders, squeezing for a peak contraction at the top. Lower under control to the start position.

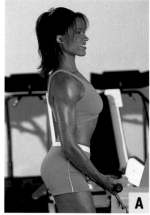

A B

Supinating Dumbbell Curl

Stand erect with your feet shoulder-width apart, holding a dumbbell in each hand using a neutral grip so the weights face your thighs. Pin your elbows to your sides, then squeeze one biceps and bend that elbow to curl one dumbbell toward your shoulder, turning your wrist as you go so your palm faces up at the top. Return under control to the start, then begin the next rep with the other arm.

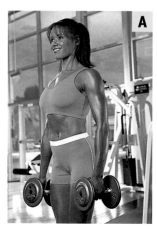

A B

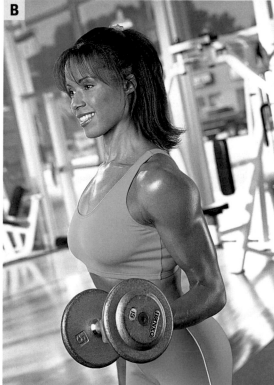

Biceps Routine

Exercise	Sets	Reps
Barbell Curl	2–3	10–12
Standing Cable Curl	2–3	10–12
Supinating Dumbbell Curl	2–3	10–12*

*each arm

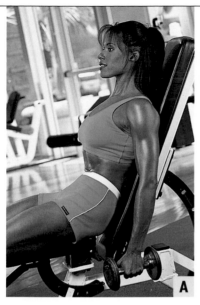
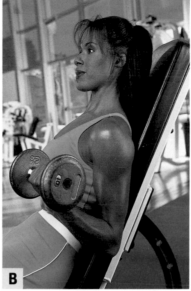

Incline Alternating Dumbbell Curl

Adjust an incline bench to about a 60-degree angle and sit with your hips and back fully supported. Grasp a dumbbell in each hand and let your arms hang straight down from your shoulders. Alternate curling the weights toward your shoulders, keeping your elbows close to the backpad throughout.

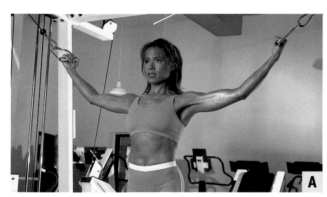

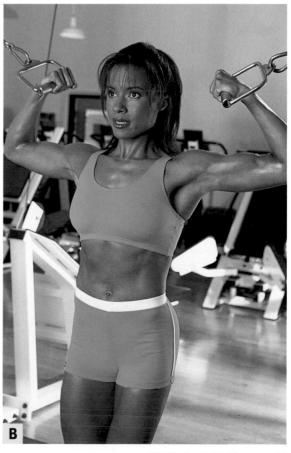

High-Cable Curl

Attach stirrup handles to both upper-pulley cables and stand in the middle of the station, torso erect, knees bent slightly and feet shoulder-width apart. Allow the resistance of the cables to pull your arms up and out to your sides so your upper arms are roughly parallel to the floor. With your palms up, squeeze both biceps to curl the handles toward your head, keeping your upper arms stationary. Release under control back to the start position.

Biceps Routine

Exercise	Sets	Reps
EZ-Bar Preacher Curl	2–3	10–12
Incline Alternating Dumbbell Curl	2–3	10–12*
High-Cable Curl	2–3	to failure

*each arm

GETTING STARTED | Making up about two-thirds of your upper-arm mass, the tri's can be a major trouble spot for women. Overtraining the muscle isn't the key, but a little confusion may do it some good. Use this at-home routine to tweak your triceps training.

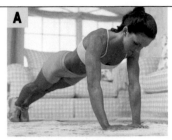

Close-Grip Push-Up

Do this one first since it's the hardest of these four exercises. Get down on your hands and knees so your arms and body are nearly perpendicular. Your hands should make a diamond shape on the floor using your thumbs and forefingers. With your abs tight and your back completely flat, slowly lower yourself until your nose almost touches the floor, then push back up to the start position. Look about 6 inches in front of you to keep your neck aligned with your back (don't flex your neck forward). For more of a challenge, come up onto your toes, as shown.

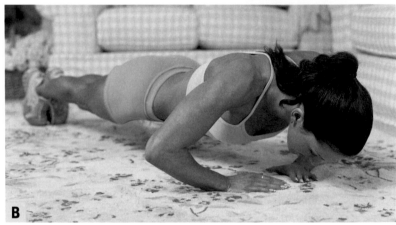

One-Arm Overhead Dumbbell Extension

This exercise can be done with both arms or one arm at a time, as shown. Sit erect with your shoulders rolled back and down. Grasp a dumbbell by cupping the inside of one plate. Extend your arm overhead, squeeze at the top, then bend your elbow to bring the weight down behind your head under control. Make sure your elbow points upward and your upper arm stays over your ear throughout the exercise. Repeat for reps, then switch sides.

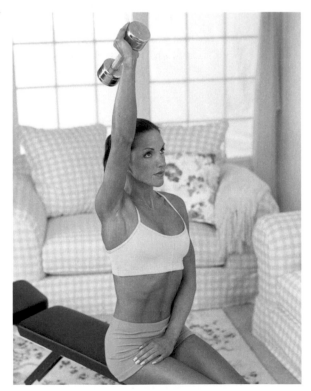

At-Home Triceps Routine

Exercise	Sets	Reps
Close-Grip Push-Up	3	10–15
One-Arm Overhead Dumbbell Extension	3	10–15*
Lying Dumbbell Extension	3	10–15
Side-Lying Push-Up	3	to failure*

*each arm

Lying Dumbbell Extension

Lie faceup on a flat bench with dumbbells in hand, palms facing in. Raise your arms straight up, then hinge at the shoulders to bring them to roughly a 45-degree angle; this is the start position. Bend your elbows to bring the weights behind your head, then squeeze your tri's to return to the start.

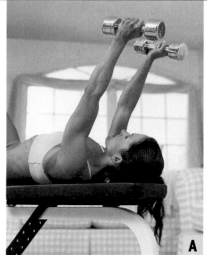 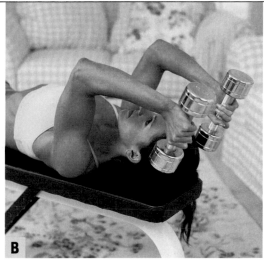

A **B**

Side-Lying Push-Up

Lie on your left side with your left arm across your abs. Place your right hand on the floor just in front of you so your elbow forms a right angle. Press through your right arm until it's nearly straight, lifting your left arm completely off the floor. Slowly lower back to the start position. Repeat to failure, then switch sides.

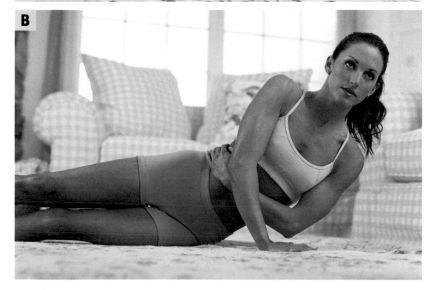

A

B

>>tip

Do a triceps workout twice a week using the exercises shown here. Each time, change the moves and the order in which you do them to confuse — and stimulate — the muscle.

GETTING STARTED | Bodyweight movements can be just as effective as weighted exercises in the gym. The bench dip and close-grip push-up are common triceps moves. Utilizing all forms of exercise at your disposal sculpts and strengthens a balanced physique.

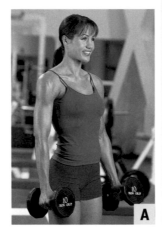
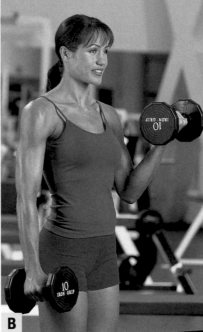

Supinating Dumbbell Curl

Stand erect with your knees slightly bent, feet shoulder-width apart. Hold dumbbells with a neutral grip (palms facing your thighs) and keep your elbows close to your sides. As you curl one or both weights toward your shoulders, slowly turn your wrists out so your palms face up in the top position. Lower under control, turning your hands back in.

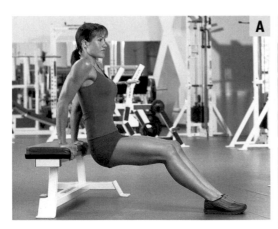
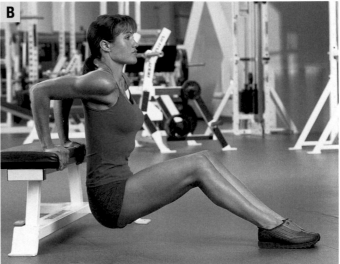

Bench Dip

Sit erect at the long edge of a bench with your feet flat on the floor. Grasp the bench just outside your hips, palms down. Move your glutes a few inches away from the bench, lower yourself under control until your elbows form 90-degree angles, then press back up. To increase the difficulty, put your feet up on a second bench.

Beginner's Arm Routine

Exercise	Sets	Reps
Supinating Dumbbell Curl	2	10–15*
Bench Dip	2	10–15
Hammer Curl	2	10–15
Straight-Bar Pressdown	2	10–15

*each arm

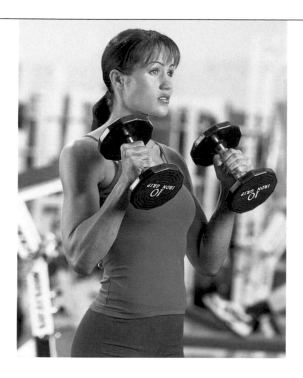

Hammer Curl

Stand erect with your knees slightly bent, feet about hip-width apart. Hold dumbbells alongside your thighs with a neutral grip (palms facing in). Keep your elbows close to your sides as you curl one or both dumbbells straight up toward your shoulders. Lower under control.

For the ultimate tank-top prep, pair this routine with Workout 31. Training arms and shoulders together in one day can ensure that these bodyparts get the attention they deserve — in and out of the gym.

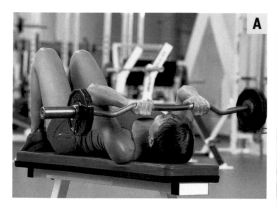

A

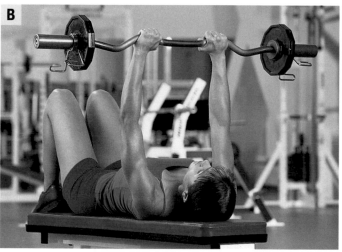

B

Lying EZ-Bar Extension

Lie faceup on a flat bench and hold an EZ-bar over your upper chest with your arms straight. Bending only your elbows, slowly lower the bar toward your forehead, stopping before it touches your head. Then contract your triceps to push the bar back up to the start position.

Intermediate Arm Routine

Exercise	Sets	Reps
Supinating Dumbbell Curl	3	10–15*
Lying EZ-Bar Extension	3	10–15
Hammer Curl	3	10–15
Bench Dip	3	10–15

*each arm

GETTING STARTED | How you train arms should depend on your goals. If you have time to give biceps and triceps a day of their own, that's the best way to add size. It's difficult to stimulate them optimally if they're already fatigued from a back or chest workout.

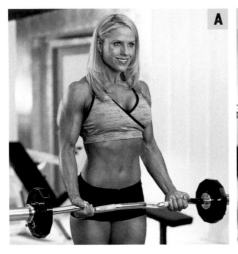
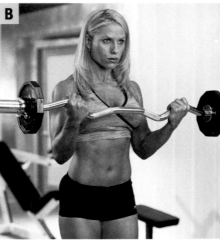

A B

EZ-Bar Curl

This exercise belongs in everyone's repertoire. It's a standard because it works, and it's comfortable to perform. Take a hip-width stance, knees slightly bent, bar down in front of your thighs. Curl the weight up while keeping your upper arms in place alongside your torso. At the top, concentrate on getting a good squeeze before lowering the bar under control. Don't lock out your elbows at the bottom.

Seated High-Cable Curl

This is a great exercise to do every once in a while for variety. Grasp a straight bar attached to the upper-pulley cable and sit on a flat bench facing the cable stack, feet planted on the floor in front of you. Keep your torso erect and upper arms stable, elbows pointing forward. Curl the bar toward your head, squeeze your biceps hard and slowly return to the start position.

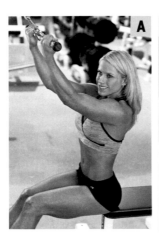

A B

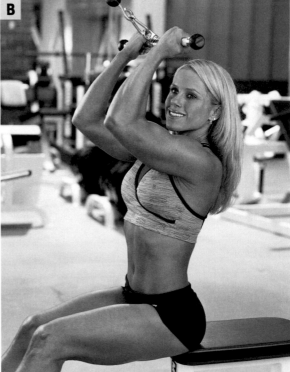

Biceps Routine

Exercise	Sets	Reps
EZ-Bar Curl	3–4	10–12
Seated High-Cable Curl	3–4	10–12
Standing Cable Concentration Curl	3–4	10–12*
*each arm		

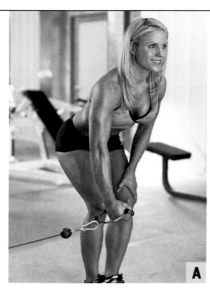

A

Standing Cable Concentration Curl

This is simply a standing version of your basic concentration curl, using the stirrup handle attached to the low-pulley cable. Stand at an angle to the cable stack, bending your knees a bit and leaning forward from your hips. Rest your outside, nonworking hand on your thigh for support. Your working arm is directly in line with your inside leg in the start position. Keeping your upper arm stationary, pull the handle straight up and across your body, squeeze at the top, then lower under control to the start. Repeat for reps, then switch sides.

>>**tip**

When using cables, stand or sit far enough away from the weight stack so there's no slack in the cable at the start of the movement.

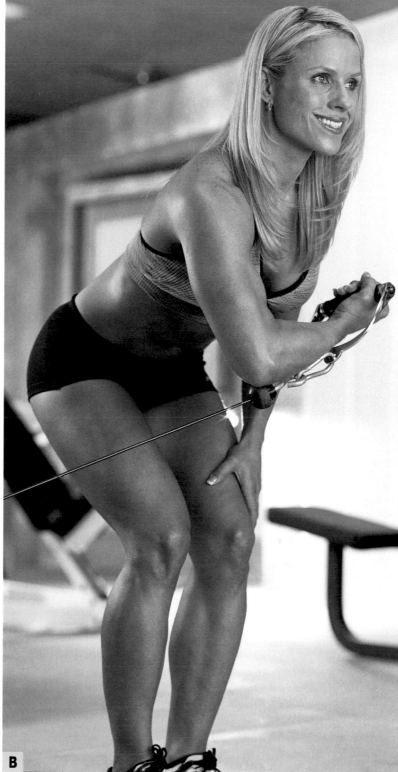

B

GETTING STARTED | The key to better biceps is positioning your body correctly. Keep your knees under your hips and slightly bent, abs pulled in and shoulders back. Try tilting your pelvis up slightly to reduce the risk of using momentum to curl the weight.

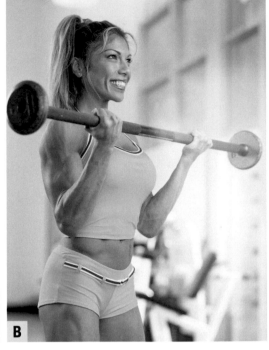

Barbell Curl

With your feet shoulder-width apart and your knees slightly bent, take a shoulder-width grip on the bar and contract your bi's to curl it up using a slow, controlled movement. Keep your chest lifted, your wrists locked and your elbows by your sides. At the top, pause for a second and squeeze your bi's, then make a conscious effort to slow down on the negative. Before your arms lock out at the bottom, pause briefly and reverse direction.

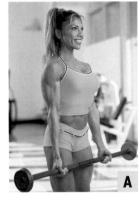

A   B

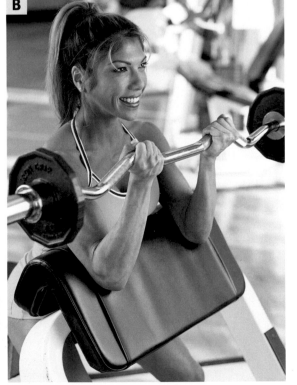

B

A

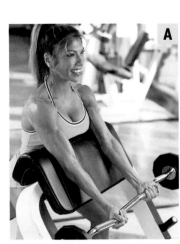

EZ-Bar Preacher Curl

Using an EZ-bar angles your wrists slightly and the bench stabilizes your arms when you position yourself so the pad supports most of your upper arms. Curl the weight up to where your elbows form roughly 90-degree angles, then lower it using a slow, controlled movement. Don't lock out; keep a slight bend in your elbows at the bottom. Make sure you lock your wrists to prevent flexing them as you bring the weight up, which would take some of the emphasis off the biceps.

Seated Alternating Dumbbell Curl

Using an upright bench for this exercise enhances stability and helps you maintain strict form. Sit erect on the bench, arms down by your sides, palms facing forward. Curl one dumbbell at a time, keeping your elbows close to your sides and turning each wrist out slightly as you squeeze your biceps at the top. Keep the movement slow and controlled as you return to the start position, then repeat with the opposite arm.

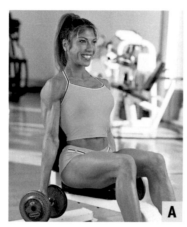
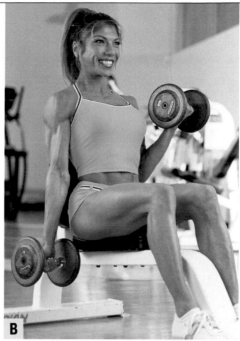

A **B**

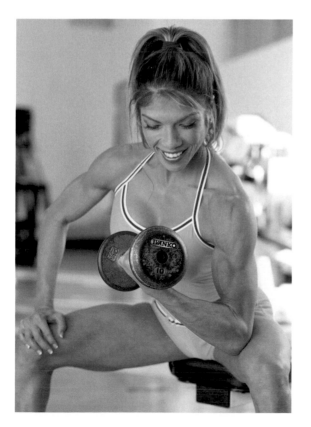

Concentration Curl

Sit erect at the end of a flat bench with your legs apart, feet flat on the floor, and bend forward from your hips. Your working arm should hang straight down from your shoulder, just touching the inside of your leg right above the knee. Keep your elbow bent slightly at the start. Curl and lower the weight using a steady, controlled pace, then switch sides.

Free-Weight Biceps Routine

Exercise	Sets	Reps
Barbell Curl	3	12–15
EZ-Bar Preacher Curl	3	12–15
Seated Alternating Dumbbell Curl	3	12–15*
Concentration Curl	3	12–15*

*each arm

GETTING STARTED | If you do the same arm workout time and again, you may not notice much improvement. Use these two workouts to progress. Start with the Beginner's Routine for 6–8 weeks. As it becomes easier, switch to the Intermediate Routine to amp up the intensity.

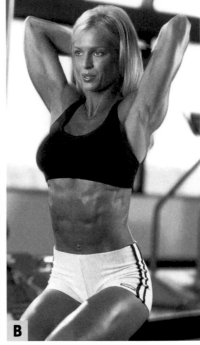

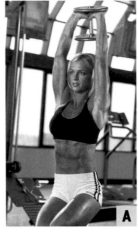

A **B**

Seated Overhead Dumbbell Extension

Use a flat bench or a seat that provides some back support but still allows for a full range of motion. Firmly cupping the inner plate of a dumbbell with both hands, lift the weight overhead to the start position, slightly retracting your shoulder blades. Keep your shoulders and arms back. Lower the weight behind your head, keeping your elbows close to your ears and getting a good stretch. Squeeze your triceps to reverse the movement and contract the muscles hard at the top.

>>tip

Increase your workout intensity by supersetting two or more exercises for the same or opposite muscle groups. Do your sets for each move back-to-back with no rest in between.

Standing Dumbbell Curl

Stand erect with your elbows fixed at your sides, then contract your biceps to curl both weights toward your shoulders. For maximum intensity, squeeze even harder at the top. Don't lock out your elbows at the bottom. You can substitute alternating dumbbell curls for this bilateral option, or try holding one dumbbell in the top position while you curl the other.

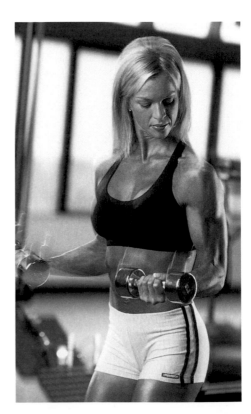

Beginner's Arm Routine

Exercise	Sets	Reps
Seated Overhead Dumbbell Extension	3	12
Straight-Bar Pressdown	3	15
EZ-Bar Curl	3	12
Standing Dumbbell Curl	3	15

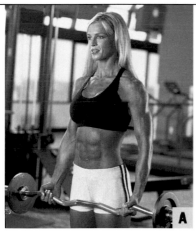

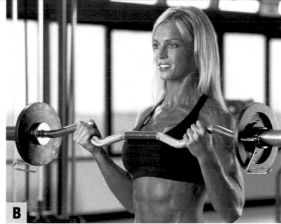

EZ-Bar Curl

Stand erect with a slight bend in your knees for stability, holding an EZ-bar with an underhand grip just outside shoulder width. Curl the bar up, squeezing your biceps hard at the top, then lower to a few inches in front of your thighs to keep tension on the muscles.

Straight-Bar Pressdown

Stand erect in front of the cable station with your knees slightly bent, grasping a straight bar attached to the upper-pulley cable just outside shoulder width. Squeeze your triceps as you press the bar to full extension, then return slowly to chest height. To emphasize the triceps rather than involve other bodyparts such as the shoulders, keep your back straight and your upper arms pinned to your sides.

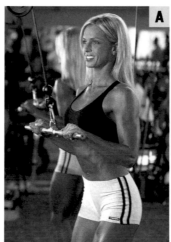

Intermediate Arm Routine

Exercise	Sets	Reps
Seated Overhead Dumbbell Extension —superset with—	5	8, 8, 6, 6, 6
Straight-Bar Pressdown	5	12, 12, 15, 15, 15
EZ-Bar Curl —superset with—	4	8, 8, 6, 6
Standing Dumbbell Curl	4	12, 12, 15, 15

Use a fairly heavy weight for low reps for the first exercise in each pairing, followed by a lighter weight for higher reps for the second exercise. Rest 1–2 minutes between supersets.

GETTING STARTED | Because the biceps and triceps are often stimulated by everyday activities such as carrying groceries or small children, you may need to use more resistance or new exercises to shock them into growth. Don't be afraid to train with heavy weights.

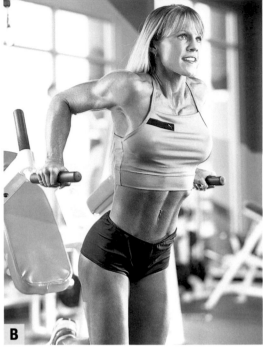

Triceps Dip

At the dip station, hold your body upright with both arms fully extended, ankles crossed behind you. Bend your elbows and descend to where your upper arms are about parallel to the bars. Don't let your shoulders fall below your elbows to avoid straining your shoulders and pecs. Push back up and slightly forward without popping your elbows; it's a soft lock at the top. Use a slightly slower pace to really feel the triceps work.

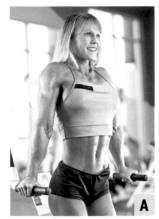

A   B

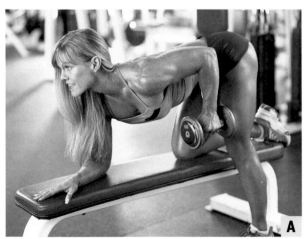

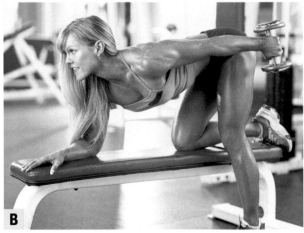

A   B

Dumbbell Kickback

To add a twist to this popular triceps-shaper, rest your nonworking forearm, not just your hand, on the bench. The slight incline keeps extra tension on the muscle throughout the exercise. With the elbow of your working arm at a right angle and close by your side, extend your arm all the way back. Keep your wrist fixed and concentrate on squeezing your triceps, not just throwing the weight back. Return to the start position slowly, resisting momentum. Repeat for reps, then switch sides.

Advanced Arm Routine

Exercise	Sets	Reps
Triceps Dip	3	20–30
Dumbbell Kickback	3	15–20*
Machine Preacher Curl	2–3	15
Hammer Curl	2	15–20

*each arm

Machine Preacher Curl

To prevent hyperextending your elbows, use a non-traditional stance: Kneel on the bench and lean into the pad, taking an underhand grip on the machine's handles. Contract your biceps to lift the weight, squeezing out a peak contraction at the top; lower it slowly, keeping a slight bend in your elbows at the bottom. Keep your elbows stationary and in line with your shoulders, your wrists straight and your grip firm but not too tight.

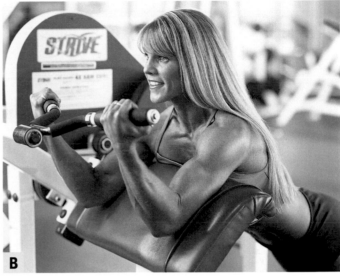

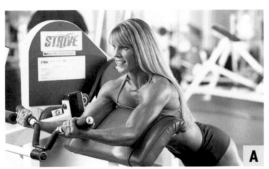

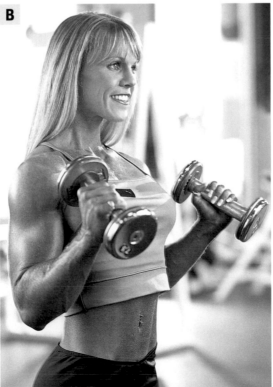

Hammer Curl

Grasp a pair of dumbbells just inside the inner plates, which will help with control. Standing erect with your knees slightly bent, arms down at your sides and palms facing in, bring the top plate of each dumbbell all the way to your shoulders, keeping your elbows down and in place at your sides. Squeeze at the top, then return to the start. You can do these simultaneously or alternate arms.

GETTING STARTED | Add these workouts to your arm arensal to really tax your muscles. Choose heavier loads for the exercises with lower rep counts and lighter loads for those with higher rep counts; in each case, you should reach failure on the last rep.

Progressive Biceps Routine

Exercise	MONTH 1 Sets	Reps	MONTH 2 Sets	Reps	MONTH 3 Sets	Reps
EZ-Bar Curl	3	8–10	3	10–12	3	12–15
Incline Dumbbell Curl	3	8–10			3	12–15
Hammer Curl			3	10–12	3	12–15*

*Do a drop set on the final set, reducing the weight by about 25% after you reach muscle failure and continuing to do as many more reps as you can.

Progressive Triceps Routine

Exercise	MONTH 1 Sets	Reps	MONTH 2 Sets	Reps	MONTH 3 Sets	Reps
Lying EZ-Bar Extension	3	8–10	3	10–12	3	12–15
Straight-Bar/Rope Pressdown	3	8–10			3	12–15
Seated Overhead Dumbbell Extension			3	10–12	3	12–15*

*Do a drop set on the final set, reducing the weight by about 25% after you reach muscle failure and continuing to do as many more reps as you can.

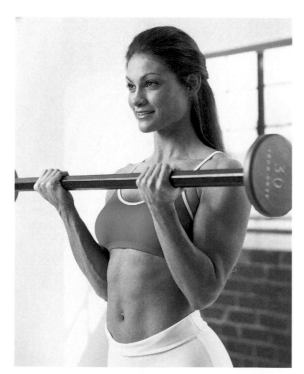

Barbell Curl

Standing erect with your feet shoulder-width apart and knees slightly bent, grasp the bar with a shoulder-width grip and contract your bi's to curl it toward your shoulders. Keep your elbows by your sides. At the top, pause and squeeze your bi's, then slow down on the return.

Right-to-Bare-Arms Routine

Exercise	Sets	Reps
BICEPS		
Standing Cable Curl	2	15 (warm-up)
EZ-Bar Curl	3	10–15
Concentration Curl	3	10–15*
Hammer Curl	3	10–15*
TRICEPS		
Reverse-Grip Straight-Bar Pressdown	2	15 (warm-up)
Lying Dumbbell Extension	3	10–15
Bench Dip	3	10–15
Dumbbell Kickback	3	10–15*

*each arm

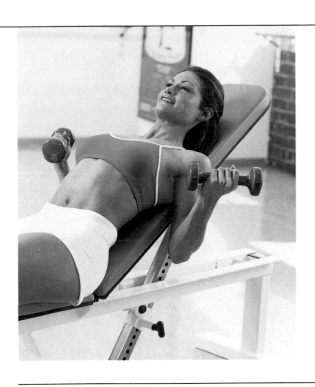

Strong-Armed Routine

Exercise	Sets	Reps
Barbell Curl	3	6
Triceps Dip	2	12
Machine Preacher Curl	3	8
Close-Grip Push-Up	3	10

Incline Dumbbell Curl

Adjust an incline bench to about a 45–60-degree angle and sit with your hips and back fully supported. Grasp a dumbbell in each hand and let your arms hang straight down from your shoulders. Simultaneously curl the weights toward your shoulders, keeping your elbows close to the backpad of the bench throughout.

>>tip

Stick with a particular workout or program for 6–8 weeks at most, then try a new routine for the same amount of time. This will keep your muscles from adapting, which can halt your progress.

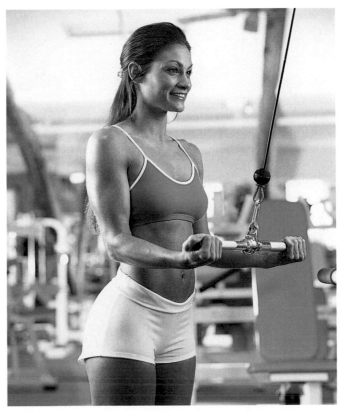

Reverse-Grip Straight-Bar Pressdown

Stand erect while facing an upper-pulley cable station, feet about hip-width apart and knees slightly bent. Grasp the short, straight bar with a shoulder-width, underhand grip and start with your forearms parallel to the floor. With your elbows tucked in close to your sides, press the bar down, moving only at the elbows until just short of locking out. Return to the start position under control.

delts

Chapter THREE

Stellar Shoulders

Optimal physical fitness starts at the top. Shapely, nicely rounded deltoids — after the Greek word *delta* that describes their triangular shape — give the appearance of a slim waistline and hips, visually balancing out any woman's physique.

GETTING STARTED | Women tend to focus on their trouble spots: thighs, midsection and backside. Yet by increasing the size and shape of your shoulders, you can change the proportions of your physique and appear more symmetrical from head to toe.

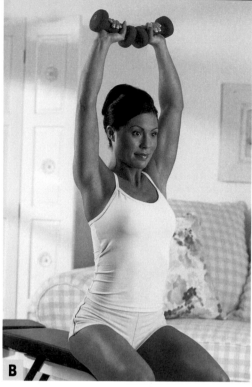

Seated Overhead Dumbbell Press

Sit erect at the end of a bench or chair, with your back supported if possible, holding dumbbells at ear level with your palms forward. Push the weights overhead by straightening your arms, but keep your elbows soft at the top. Keep control over the weights; don't let them bang together. Return to the arms-parallel position.

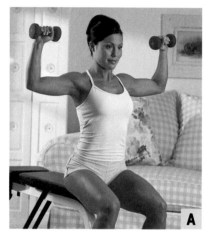

A B

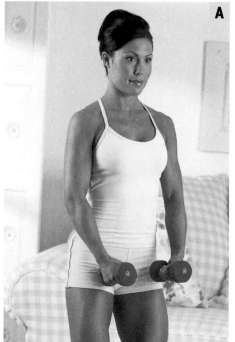

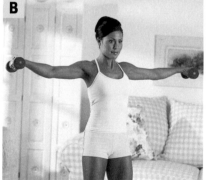

A B

Lateral Raise

Stand erect with your feet shoulder-width apart, knees slightly bent. Hold dumbbells in front of your thighs with your palms facing in and your elbows bent slightly. Lift the weights up and out to shoulder level while keeping that slight bend in your elbows. For maximum contraction, your wrists, elbows and shoulders should be aligned at the top. Control the descent.

At-Home Shoulder Routine

Exercise	Sets	Reps
Seated Overhead Dumbbell Press	3	12–15
Lateral Raise	3	12–15
Dumbbell Upright Row —superset with—	3	12–15
Bent-Over Lateral Raise	3	12–15

To perform a superset, do your reps for each exercise back-to-back with no rest in between.

Dumbbell Upright Row

Stand erect and grasp a pair of dumbbells in front of you with your hands just inside shoulder-width apart, palms facing your body. Pull the weights up while keeping them close to your body, leading with your elbows, until your hands are just beneath your shoulders. In the finish position, your elbows should be higher than your wrists and above the level of your shoulders. Release slowly and under control.

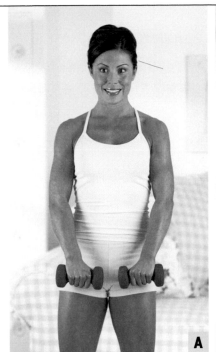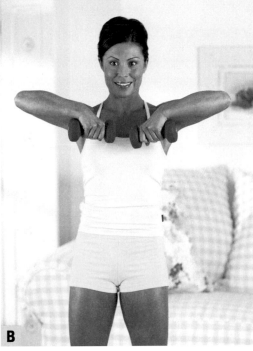

A   **B**

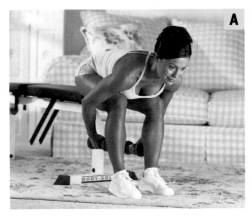

A   **B**

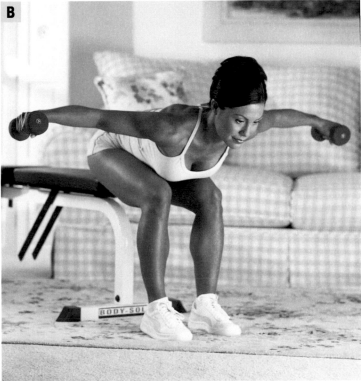

Bent-Over Lateral Raise

Sit at the end of a bench and bend forward at your hips so your chest is as close to your thighs as is comfortable. Hold dumbbells under your legs with your palms facing each other and your elbows slightly bent. Keep your head neutral by looking at a spot on the floor that's about 6 inches in front of your feet. Focus on using your rear delts to lift the weights out to your sides to shoulder level while keeping that slight bend in your elbows. Return following the same arc.

GETTING STARTED | In general, training your shoulders once a week should be enough to see results. If yours seem to be particularly stubborn, however, try training them twice a week, alternating between heavy and light workouts, for about a month.

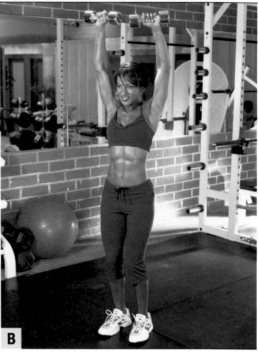

Standing Overhead Dumbbell Press

With a dumbbell in each hand, stand erect with your feet about hip-width apart. Lift the weights to ear level, elbows bent and pointing toward the floor, palms facing forward. Extend your arms to press the dumbbells overhead, stopping short of locking your elbows. Keep your shoulders down by squeezing your shoulder blades together. Follow the same arcing path on the descent.

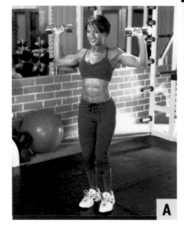

A **B**

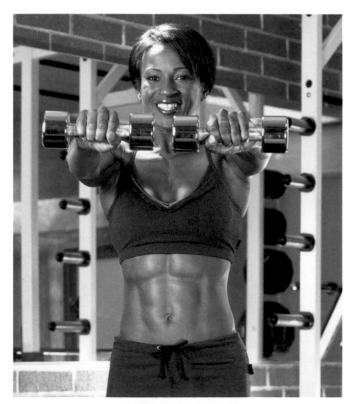

Front Dumbbell Raise

With a dumbbell in each hand in front of your thighs, stand erect with your feet about hip-width apart and knees slightly bent. Keep a slight arch in your back, abs tight, shoulders squared and eyes directed forward. Raise the dumbbells straight out in front of you until your arms are parallel to the floor, just above shoulder height. Pause for a moment, then return to the start.

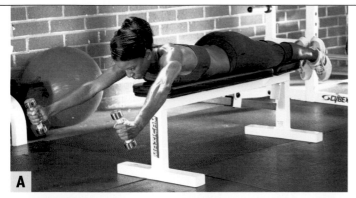

A

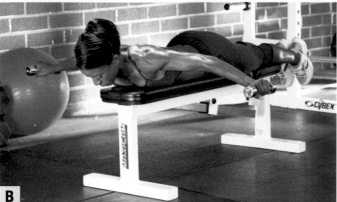

B

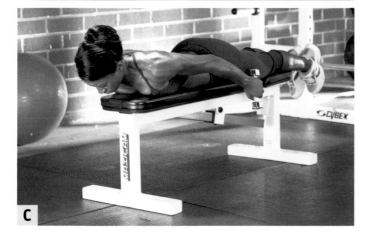

C

Y, T & I

This exercise strengthens the rotator cuff and is helpful in preventing shoulder impingement syndrome. Grasp two very light dumbbells and lie facedown on a flat bench, letting your arms hang straight down off the sides. Rotate your thumbs up to lead the way. Squeeze your shoulder blades together and lift both arms toward your head to form the letter "Y" (A); slowly lower and repeat for reps. Next, let your arms hang straight down off the bench with your palms facing each other. Squeeze your shoulder blades together and raise your arms out to your sides to form the letter "T" (B); lower and repeat for reps. Last, start with your arms hanging down off the bench, thumbs pointing down. Lift your arms behind you, keeping them as close to your body as possible, to form the letter "I" (C); lower and repeat for reps.

Dumbbell Shoulder Routine

Exercise	Sets	Reps
Standing Overhead Dumbbell Press	2	12–15
Front Dumbbell Raise	2	12–15
Y, T & I	2	12–15

>>tip

To continue making progress, change the variables of your workout each time. You can choose different exercises, change the order in which you do them, or vary your equipment and weight loads.

GETTING STARTED | Delts are commonly referred to by their three sections — the front, middle and rear deltoids. This at-home routine groups four exercises in supersets to provide a complete workout, training all three heads of the shoulder with a challenging twist.

Upright Row

Place the resistance band securely under your heels and stand erect with your feet slightly apart. Hold one handle in each hand, palms facing your thighs, arms extended. Leading with your elbows, lift your hands until they come to just under your chin. Your elbows should be higher than your hands in the top position. Lower slowly to full arm extension. Repeat for reps; without resting, adjust your position and begin the alternating lateral and front raise.

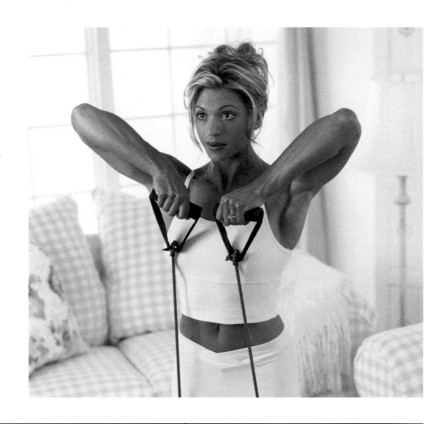

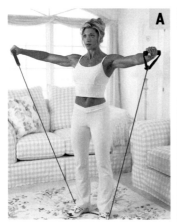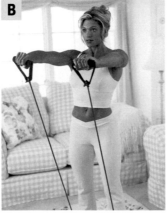

Alternating Lateral and Front Raise

With a handle in each hand and your arms down at your sides, soften your elbows and press your shoulders down and back. Keeping your spine and lower back completely still, lift the handles out to each side to the 3 and 9 o'clock positions (A). Pause for a moment before returning to the start. For the second part of the rep, lift the handles out in front of you so your arms are in line with your shoulders (B). Alternate lateral and front raises.

One-Arm Bent-Over Lateral Raise

Stand in a lunge position with your right foot on the band, grasping the handle with your right hand, palm facing in. Keeping your back flat, bend from the hips so that your back and left leg make almost a straight line. Support your position with your left hand on a chair or your leg. Lift your right arm straight out to your side until it's parallel to the floor. Repeat for reps; without resting, adjust your position and begin the one-arm overhead press.

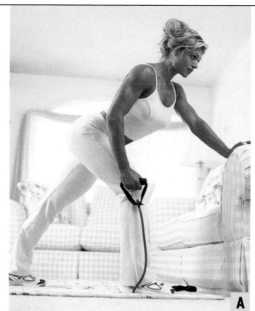 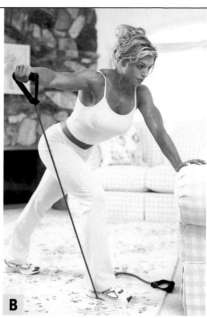

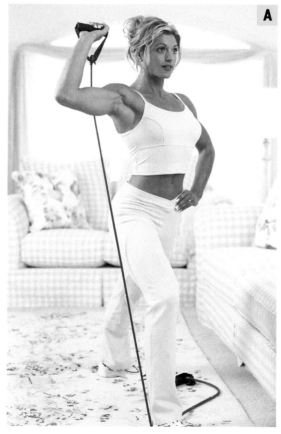 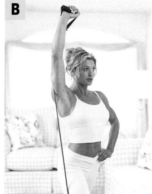

One-Arm Overhead Press

Stand erect in a slight lunge position, right heel on the band. Start with your left hand on your hip and your right hand slightly above and next to your shoulder, palm forward. Holding the handle securely with the band running behind your arm, extend your arm overhead without locking out your elbow. Slowly return to the start position. Repeat for reps and switch sides.

Resistance-Band Routine

Exercise	Sets	Reps
Upright Row —superset with—	3	10–12
Alternating Lateral and Front Raise	3	12–15 each
One-Arm Bent-Over Lateral Raise —superset with—	3	12–15*
One-Arm Overhead Press	3	12–15*

To perform a superset, do your reps for each exercise back-to-back with no rest in between.
*each side

GETTING STARTED | Shoulders can end up taking a backseat to the larger muscle groups, especially when you train chest or back first in your workout. Try training your delts first, when your strength and energy levels are high, to give them priority.

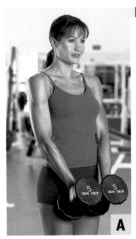
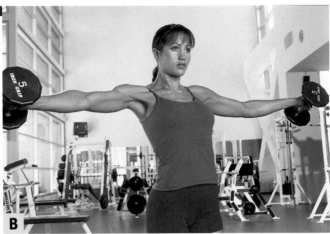

Lateral Raise

Stand erect with your knees slightly bent, abs contracted and feet shoulder-width apart. Hold the dumbbells in front of your thighs with your palms facing in, elbows slightly bent. Leading with your elbows, raise your arms up and out to your sides in an arc till they come parallel to the floor. Lower under control.

Seated Overhead Dumbbell Press

Sit erect on a bench with a back support, holding dumbbells at about ear level so your upper arms are roughly parallel to the floor, elbows close to 90 degrees. Press the dumbbells overhead in a slight arc until your arms are straight but not locked out, then lower under control.

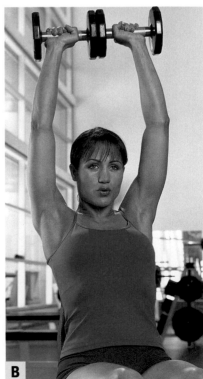
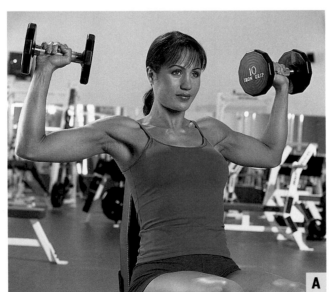

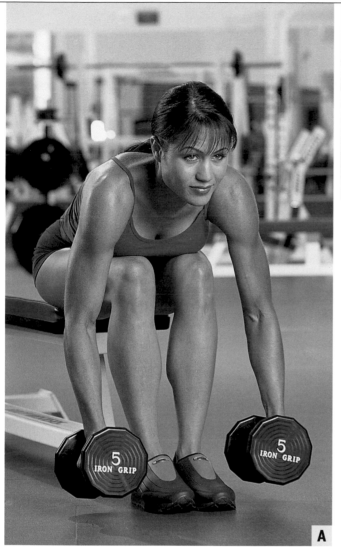

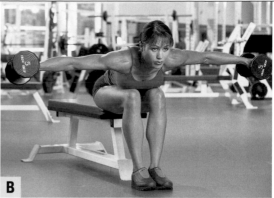

Bent-Over Lateral Raise

With dumbbells in hand, sit at the end of a flat bench with your feet and knees together. Bend forward at the hips so your chest touches your thighs, allowing the dumbbells to hang down alongside your legs. Keep a slight bend in your elbows as you raise your arms up and out to your sides in an arc, stopping when they're about parallel to the floor. Lower under control.

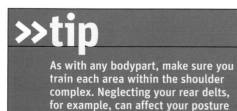

>>tip

As with any bodypart, make sure you train each area within the shoulder complex. Neglecting your rear delts, for example, can affect your posture and even put you at risk for injury.

Dumbbell Shoulder Routine

Exercise	Sets	Reps
Lateral Raise	2–3	10–15
Seated Overhead Dumbbell Press	2–3	10–15
Bent-Over Lateral Raise	2–3	10–15

GETTING STARTED | The key to strong and shapely shoulders is a workout that targets all three deltoid heads. This routine focuses on the middle head to sculpt the tops and sides of the shoulders, with the cheerleader move pulling double-duty on the front and rear delts.

Standing Overhead Dumbbell Press

Stand erect with dumbbells in hand, elbows bent 90 degrees and raised to ear level, palms forward, knees slightly bent and abs tight. Press the weights up and toward each other as you straighten your arms, keeping just a slight bend in your elbows at the top. Return to the start position under control.

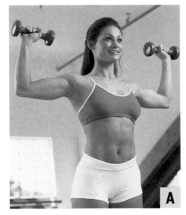
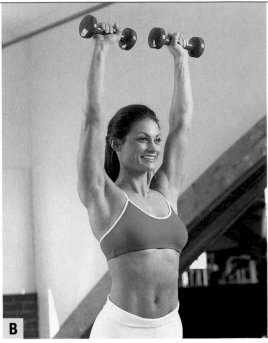

Lateral Raise

Stand erect holding dumbbells down in front of your thighs, elbows and knees slightly bent, abs tight and shoulders relaxed. Raise your arms up and out to your sides in a wide arc to about shoulder level, leading with your elbows. Slowly return to the start position.

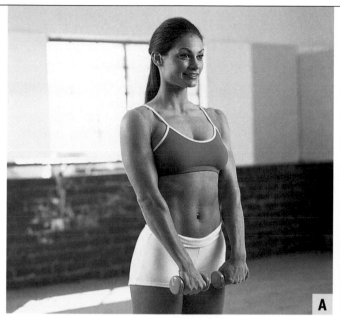
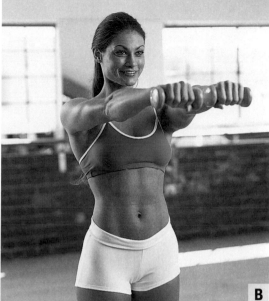
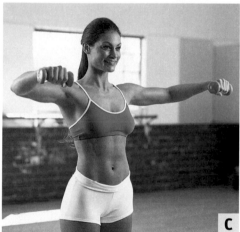
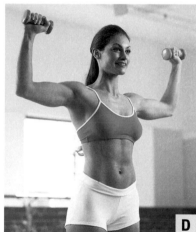
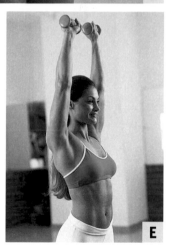

Cheerleader

Stand erect holding light dumbbells in front of your thighs, palms facing you (A). Keeping your elbows slightly bent, lift the weights to shoulder height in front of you (B). Next, bend your elbows and pull the weights back toward your shoulders, keeping your arms parallel to the floor (C). Pause, then externally rotate at the shoulders to move into the start position of an overhead press (D). Extend your arms overhead (E), then return to the start. Repeat the sequence for reps.

>>tip

When doing the cheerleader exercise, separate each position into a clean and controlled movement. Blending them together too quickly leads to sloppy form and can cause injury.

Dumbbell Shoulder Routine

Exercise	Sets	Reps
Standing Overhead Dumbbell Press	3	10–12
Lateral Raise	3	10–12
Cheerleader	2–3	10–12

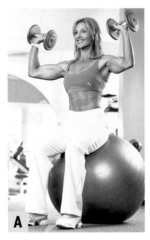
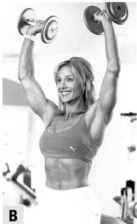
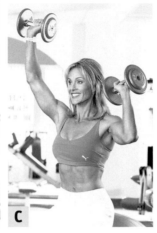

Exercise-Ball Overhead Dumbbell Press

Sit atop a ball and hold a dumbbell in each hand at shoulder level (A). Keeping your low back in its natural arch and your abs tight, press both weights overhead, allowing them to arc naturally toward each other (B). Stop when your elbows are almost straight and the dumbbells nearly touch at the top, then return the weights to shoulder level. After 15 reps, do alternating reps for another 10 per side — pressing one dumbbell up as you lower the other (C) — for the last two sets.

Reverse Cable Crossover

Stand in the center of an upper-pulley cable station and grasp the opposite handle in each hand (the left handle in your right hand and vice versa) so your hands cross in front of you at about shoulder height. With proper posture and spinal alignment from head to tailbone and keeping your elbows just slightly bent throughout, squeeze your rear delts to pull the handles out and back until your body forms a lowercase "t," then return to the start. Your elbows should point straight back as you pull the cables across your body.

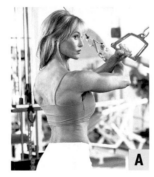
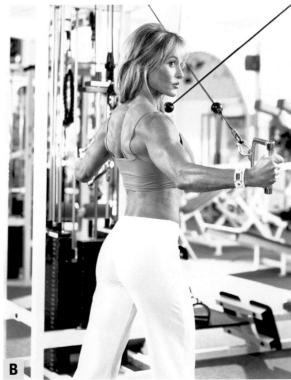

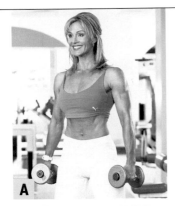

Multi-Angle Dumbbell Raise

Stand erect, grasping a dumbbell in each hand with your arms extended (A). Raise both weights in front of you, palms facing down (B). Lower them back to the start, then raise them both out to your sides (not pictured) and back down. On the third rep, raise your left hand out to your side and your right hand to the front (C), then return to the start. Finally, raise your right hand out to your side and your left hand to the front (D). Keep each of the four movements slow and strict so you don't bounce the weights up, and repeat the sequence for reps to complete a full set.

The pike push-up has multiple levels of difficulty, from keeping your legs bent (the easiest), to legs straight (shown below), to an even more advanced version where you lift one foot off the bench.

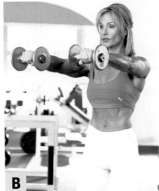

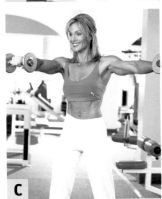

Pike Push-Up

Begin in a push-up position with your toes up on a flat bench behind you, and walk your hands in to push your hips up to a 90-degree angle in the air. Keep your legs straight and the natural curve in your low back throughout. Bend your elbows to lower yourself until your head is a few inches from the floor, elbows pointing outward as you descend. Squeeze your delts to press back up. Move slowly and under control; stop as soon as you start to lose control and break form.

A

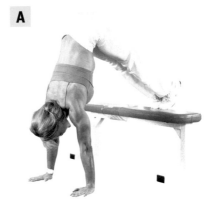

B

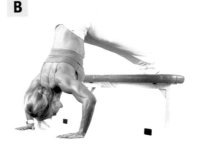

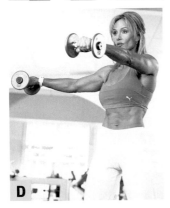

Advanced Shoulder Routine

Exercise	Sets	Reps
Exercise-Ball Overhead Dumbbell Press	3	15, 10/10, 10/10
Pike Push-Up	2–3	10
Reverse Cable Crossover	2–3	10–15
Multi-Angle Dumbbell Raise	2–3	12–16

GETTING STARTED | The shoulders get a lot of stimulation in arm, back and chest workouts, making it difficult to fully isolate the delts. Focus on the area you're training, thinking of your hands only as hooks to minimize arm involvement.

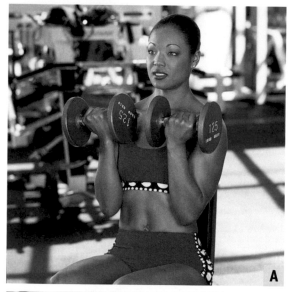

A

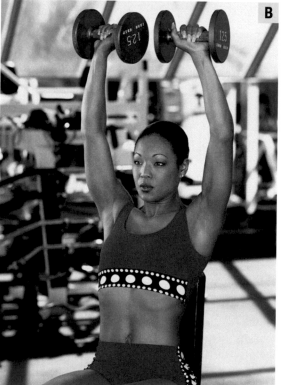

B

Shoulder-Molder Routine

Exercise	Sets	Reps
One-Arm Cable Overhead Press	5	10*
Cable Upright Row^	5	10
Lateral Raise	4	15
Bent-Over Lateral Raise	4	20

*each arm
^Perform like the dumbbell move but use a short bar attached to the low-pulley cable.

Advanced Shoulder Routine

Exercise	Sets	Reps
Arnold Press	3	12
—superset with—		
Seated Lateral Raise	3	12
Wide-Grip Barbell Upright Row^	2	15
—superset with—		
Front Barbell Raise	2	15

^Perform like the dumbbell move but use a barbell.

Strong Shoulders Routine

Exercise	Sets	Reps
Standing Military Press	3	6
Side-Lying One-Arm Lateral Raise	2	12*
One-Arm Overhead Press (with rest at top)^	3	8*

*each arm
^Perform like the seated overhead dumbbell press but start with your arms overhead and alternate reps to each side.

Arnold Press

Sit on a low-back bench holding dumbbells directly in front of your shoulders with a supinated (palms facing you) grip, elbows pointing downward. Press the weights overhead while turning your wrists so that your palms face forward at the top of the movement. Slowly lower the dumbbells along the same path.

Front Barbell Raise

Stand erect with your feet shoulder-width apart and grasp a barbell with a shoulder-width, overhand grip in front of your upper thighs. Keep your chest up, shoulders back and knees slightly bent. Keeping your arms straight, lift the barbell in a smooth motion to shoulder height. Slowly return to the start.

Standing Military Press *(not shown)*

Stand erect holding a barbell behind your neck just outside shoulder width, elbows pointing out to your sides. Squeeze your shoulders to press the bar overhead to just short of elbow lockout. Pause, then return under control.

Side-Lying One-Arm Lateral Raise *(not shown)*

Sit sideways on an incline bench set to a 45–60-degree angle, nonworking arm across your abs. Grasp a dumbbell in your outside hand, palm facing your thigh. Keeping a slight bend in your elbow, squeeze your delt to raise your arm to perpendicular to your body, then control the descent. Repeat for reps, then switch sides.

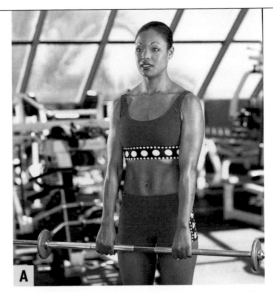

A

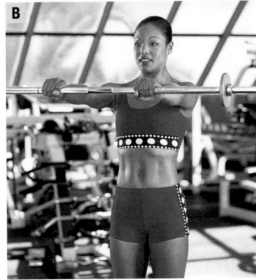

B

>>tip

When choosing weights for these exercises, pick heavier weights for lower rep ranges and lighter weights for higher rep ranges. Use heavy weights only after warming up.

Unilateral Shoulder Routine

Exercise	Sets	Reps
Exercise-Ball Overhead Dumbbell Press	3	10*
Alternating Dumbbell Lateral and Front Raise^	2–3	10 each
Y, T & I	2–3	10

*each arm
^Perform like the resistance-band move but use dumbbells.

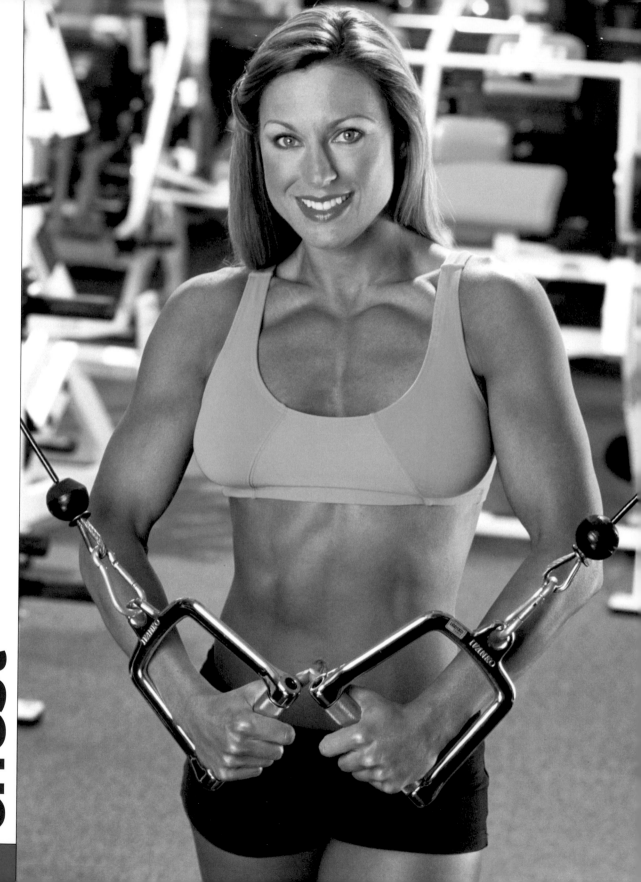

chest

Chapter FOUR

Perfect Pectorals

There's more to a head-turning physique than taut abs and thighs. As one of your largest bodyparts, the chest is vital to upper-body strength and muscular balance. Train it to its fullest in your quest to sculpt your torso.

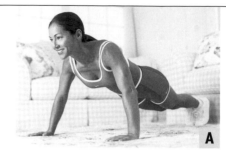

GETTING STARTED | Chest training is an important component of your upper-body strength routine. If you're new to resistance training, start with 1–2 sets of both a press and flye move, then progress gradually to three sets or add another exercise.

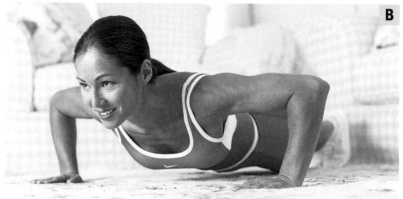

Push-Up

Lie facedown on the floor with your hands flat, slightly wider than shoulder-width apart, fingers pointing forward. Push your bodyweight off the floor by squeezing your chest and straightening your elbows, keeping your abs tight and body in a straight line, supported on your hands and toes. Bend your elbows and lower your body until your elbows form 90-degree angles and point out to the sides. Don't allow your chest to touch the floor. Pause, then contract your chest and push back up.

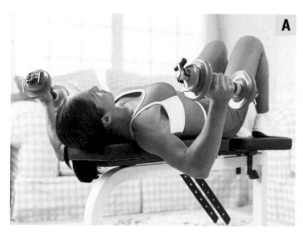

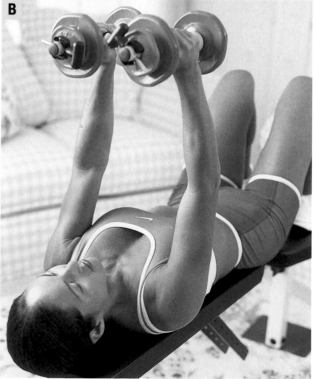

Dumbbell Flye

Lie faceup on a flat bench holding dumbbells directly above your chest with your arms almost fully extended and palms facing in. Slowly lower the weights straight out to your sides, trying to keep most of the motion in your shoulder joints, not your elbows. Lower to a point where you feel a slight stretch through your chest. Squeeze your pecs and bring the dumbbells together in an arc back to the start position.

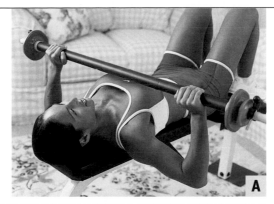

A

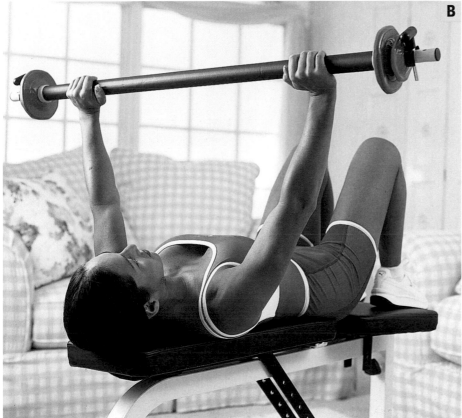

B

Barbell Bench Press

Lie faceup on a flat bench, grasp a barbell a little wider than shoulder width and hold it slightly above the center of your chest, elbows pointing out to your sides. Contract your chest to press the bar directly upward until your arms are fully extended, elbows unlocked. Slowly lower the bar back to the start position.

>>tip

Avoid arching your back or using muscle-robbing momentum to get the weight up. If you find you can't keep your form, use a lighter weight.

At-Home Chest Routine

Exercise	Sets	Reps
Push-Up	3	12–15
Barbell Bench Press	3	12–15
Dumbbell Flye	3	12–15

GETTING STARTED | Chest exercises come in two main varieties: the flye and the press. Use both as well as train from different angles. Using an incline emphasizes the upper portion of the muscle; a flat bench focuses on the center of the chest and is good for overall strength.

Dumbbell Bench Press

Lie faceup on a flat bench with your feet on the floor or up on the end of the bench. With a dumbbell in each hand near the sides of your chest, palms facing your feet, press the dumbbells up so they meet over your chest, but control the movement so they don't touch at the top. On the return, bring your elbows to just past parallel to the floor to get a slight stretch through the pecs.

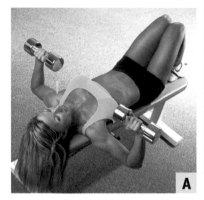

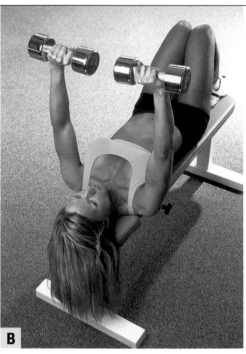

A **B**

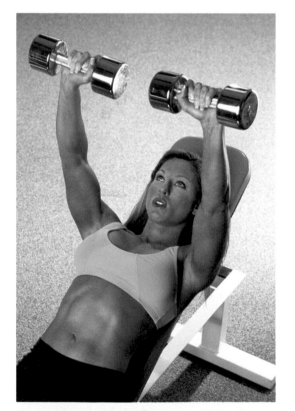

Incline Dumbbell Press

Performing a press on the incline bench requires that you align yourself and the weights properly. Lie faceup on a bench set to a 30–45-degree incline, feet on the floor, your chest arched upward and abs tight to stabilize your body. Using a similar range of motion as on a flat-bench press, press the weights directly over your upper chest and squeeze at the top, then return under full control so your upper arms dip just past parallel to the floor. Don't go any deeper or you risk injury to your shoulder joints.

≫tip

Do 2–3 light sets of your first multi-joint exercise before your working sets to warm up your shoulders and elbows. When using dumbbells, keep your elbows and shoulders in the same plane to prevent injury.

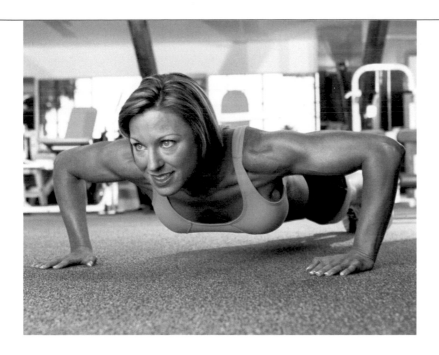

Push-Up

Get in push-up position, hands about 4 inches outside your shoulders. Contract your abs and keep your neck aligned with your spine. Stay up on your toes if you can. Keep the motion controlled, two seconds down, two seconds up. For variety, you can put your feet atop an exercise ball or bench for more of a challenge. This also changes the angle of the movement to involve more of the upper chest.

Cable Crossover

Attach stirrup handles to the upper-pulley cables. Using a split stance, stand erect in the center of the cable station with your hands directly in front of you, chest up and abs tight. Begin the movement by allowing the tension in the cables to pull your arms out to your sides and just past the plane of your body for a stretch, then squeeze your chest and push your arms forward to return to the start position, keeping your elbows slightly bent. Perform this exercise with complete control.

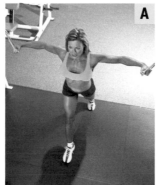

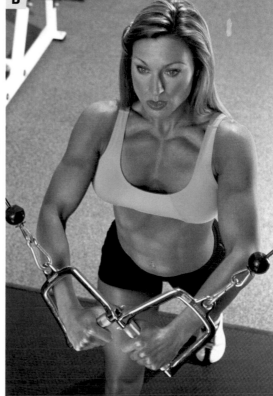

Chest Routine

Exercise	Sets	Reps
Dumbbell Bench Press	3	12–15
Incline Dumbbell Press	3	12–15
Cable Crossover	3	12–15
Push-Up	3	12–15 or to failure

GETTING STARTED | Let's face it — all women are not created equal. While you can't double your cup size through training chest alone, you may notice more muscular roundness and fullness in your pectoral muscles that enhance your natural shape.

Exercise-Ball Push-Up

Get into push-up position with the ball under your shins, hands just outside shoulder-width apart. Keep your back flat so your body forms a straight line from head to toes. Lower your head and chest only as far as your shoulder comfort permits, and don't allow your lower back to arch or your hips to sag. Remember to keep your chest lifted as you press back up. If you're a beginner, position the ball closer to your hips for more support and progressively move the ball down your legs as you become more comfortable with the exercise.

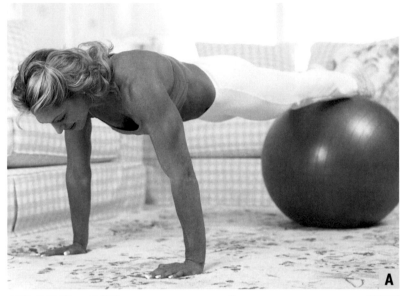

A

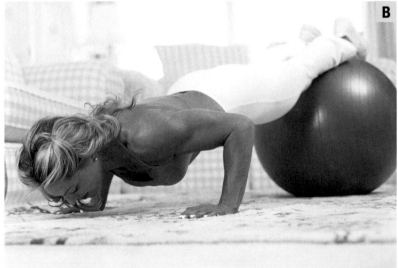

B

Beginner Option

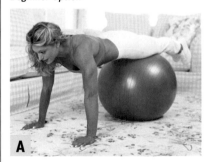

A

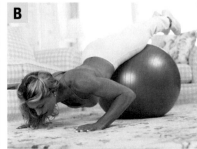

B

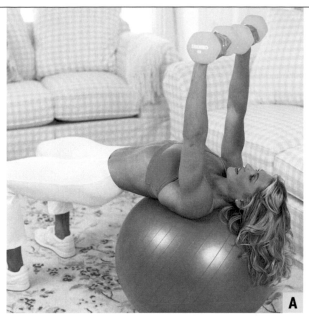

Exercise-Ball Dumbbell Press

Lie faceup atop the ball so your upper torso, neck and head are fully supported; knees are bent 90 degrees. Keep your upper body and thighs parallel to the floor. With a dumbbell in each hand just above your shoulders, palms facing your feet, squeeze your chest to extend your arms directly over your chest. Slowly return to the arms-parallel position.

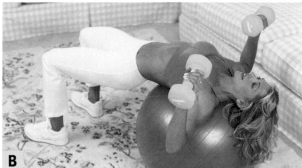

A B

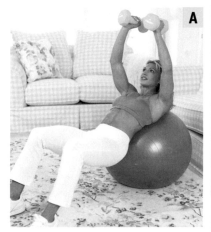

A B

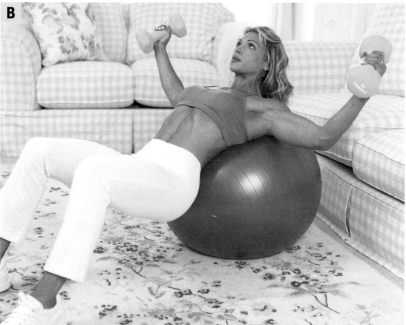

Exercise-Ball Incline Flye

Position yourself on the ball so your torso is at about a 45-degree angle to the floor. Your hips should be low, and your knees high with your feet wide and flat on the floor. Start with a dumbbell in each hand, arms extended directly over your shoulders with your palms facing each other. With your elbows slightly bent, slowly lower the weights out to your sides in an arc, stopping when your upper arms are parallel to the floor. Squeeze your chest to follow the same arc on the return.

Exercise-Ball Chest Routine

Exercise	Sets	Reps
Exercise-Ball Push-Up	3	12–15
Exercise-Ball Dumbbell Press	3	12–15
Exercise-Ball Incline Flye	3	12–15

GETTING STARTED | While most women don't have to worry about their one-arm push-up strength, gaining a bit of power in the pecs is important for muscle balance. After all, if you train back but never chest, you may be prone to shoulder injuries and posture issues.

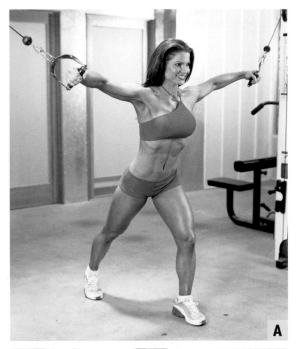

A

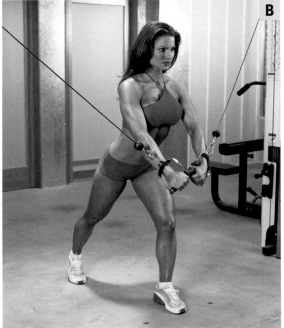

B

Cable Crossover

Attach stirrup handles to the upper-pulley cables and use an overhand grip. Stand between the stations, using a split stance and leaning slightly forward from your hips. With your arms extended out to your sides in the start position, hands just above the level of your shoulders, squeeze your pecs to pull the handles down and across your body, bringing them together in front of your abs. To increase the range of motion, cross your wrists so your palms face your body. Keep a slight bend in your elbows throughout. Slowly return to the start position.

>>tip

Rotate these machine exercises out of your routine every 4–6 weeks in favor of free-weight and bodyweight moves. This promotes complete muscle development and reduces workout boredom.

Chest Routine

Exercise	Sets	Reps
Barbell Bench Press	2–3	12–15
Cable Crossover	2–3	12–15
Machine Press	2–3	12–15
Pec-Deck Flye	2–3	12–15

Machine Press

Use a machine that places your body in an upright or incline position. Adjust the seat and visualize a straight bar going from handle to handle across your chest. Push the handles away from you, fully extending your arms without locking out your elbows. Pause and return to the start, bringing the handles about 2 inches from your body.

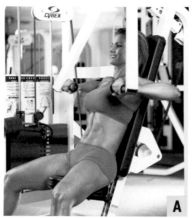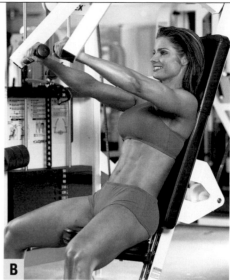

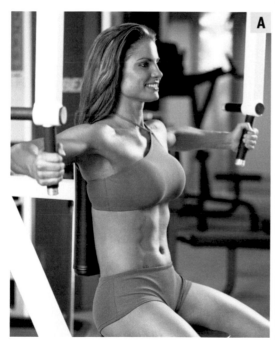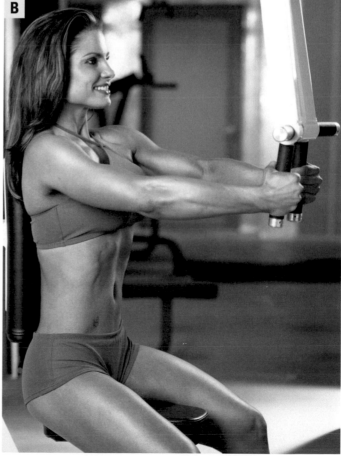

Pec-Deck Flye

Adjust the seat so your wrists, elbows and shoulders are in the same plane. Grasp the handles out to your sides with your elbows slightly bent and squeeze your pecs to bring the handles together in front of your chest. Pause, then slowly control the return. Don't break the horizontal plane or allow your elbows to move behind your shoulders.

GETTING STARTED | Swap out your usual chest routine with one of these hardcore options. Each workout will challenge your strength and add shape to your chest. Concentrate on squeezing your pecs to move the weight so your arms don't take over.

"I Love Push-Ups" Routine

Exercise	Sets	Reps
Weighted Push-Up	3	12
—superset with—		
Push-Up (without weight)	3	to failure
Exercise-Ball Push-Up	3	12–15
Medicine-Ball Push-Up (one hand on ball, one on floor)	2*	12–15

*one set per side
To perform a superset, do your reps for each exercise back-to-back with no rest in between.

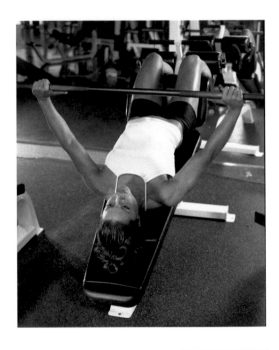

Smith-Machine Decline Press

Lie faceup on a decline bench within the Smith machine, feet under the rollers, your chest arched upward and abs tight to stabilize your body. Using a similar range of motion as on a flat-bench press, unhook the bar using a grip slightly wider than shoulder width and press it directly over your lower chest. Squeeze at the top, then return under control so your upper arms dip just past parallel to the floor.

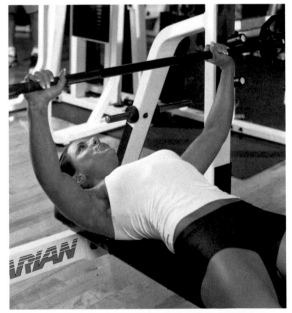

Barbell Bench Press

Lie faceup on a flat bench, grasp a barbell a little wider than shoulder width and hold it slightly above the center of your chest, elbows pointing out to your sides. Contract your chest to press the bar directly upward until your arms are fully extended, elbows unlocked. Slowly lower the bar back to the start position.

"I Love Presses" Routine

Exercise	Sets	Reps
Barbell Bench Press	3	10, 8, 6
Dumbbell Bench Press with light weights	1	to failure
Incline Barbell Press	3	8–12
—superset with—		
Smith-Machine Decline Press	3	8–12

To perform a superset, do your reps for each exercise back-to-back with no rest in between.

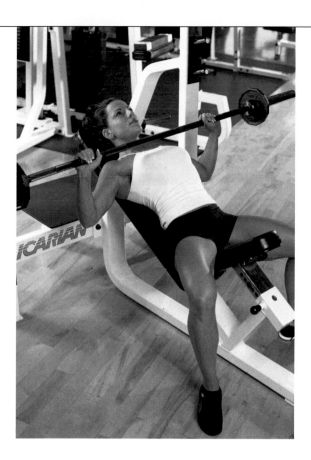

Fast & Furious Chest Routine

Exercise	Sets	Reps
Barbell Bench Press	3	8–10
Pec-Deck Flye —tri-set with—	3	15
Incline Dumbbell Press	3	15
Push-Up	3	15
Machine Press —tri-set with—	3	15
Cable Crossover	3	15
Push-Up	3	15

To perform a tri-set, do your reps for each exercise back-to-back with no rest in between.

Incline Barbell Press

Lie faceup on an incline bench set to 30–45 degrees within a rack, feet on the floor, your chest arched upward and abs tight to stabilize your body. Using a similar range of motion as on a flat-bench press, remove the bar from the rack with a grip slightly wider than shoulder width and press it directly over your upper chest. Squeeze at the top, then return under control so your upper arms dip just past parallel to the floor.

Weighted Push-Up *(not shown)*

Get in push-up position and have a spotter place a small weight plate across your upper back. Push your body-weight off the floor by straightening your elbows, keeping your abs tight and body in a straight line, supported on your hands and toes. Bend your elbows to 90-degree angles. Pause, then squeeze your chest to push back up.

Heavy-Lifting Chest Routine

Exercise	Sets	Reps
Barbell Bench Press	4	5–6
Dumbbell Bench Press	5	6
Incline Dumbbell Flye	3	8

>>tips

When training chest, remember these pointers:
>> Warm up with 1–2 lightweight sets of your first exercise.
>> Don't bounce at the bottom. Movements should be smooth and controlled to prevent injury.
>> Don't use excessively heavy weights. This forces the involvement of other muscles, such as the shoulders, core and legs. Correct technique is your priority.
>> When doing flyes and presses, stopping at the bottom position makes the exercise more difficult. Change directions quickly yet smoothly to transfer the energy from the eccentric down phase to the concentric up phase.

back

Chapter FIVE

Beautiful Back

Confidence emanates from a woman who stands tall, holding her head and chest high and her shoulders back. Our targeted workouts can help you power up your posture as you sculpt a strong and shapely rear view.

GETTING STARTED | Whether you're lifting weights for the first time or you've hit a plateau, these essential exercises should be the backbone of your training. Learn their many variations to keep your workout fresh and exciting — and your development progressing.

One-Arm Dumbbell Row

For this free-weight exercise, form is everything. Place your right hand and knee on a flat bench, grasp a dumbbell in your left hand, and keep your back flat and head in a neutral position. Pull the dumbbell up toward the side of your waist using a slow and controlled motion, keeping your elbow close to your body. Squeeze your back muscles to pull your shoulder blade toward the center of your back. Don't twist your body, or allow your back to round or your shoulders to hunch. Control the return. Repeat for reps, then switch sides.

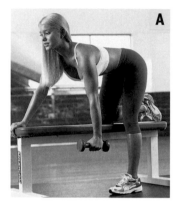
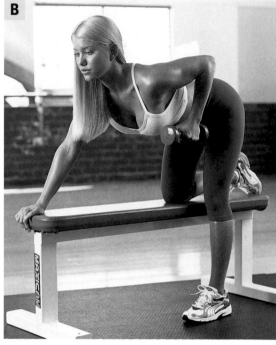

A B

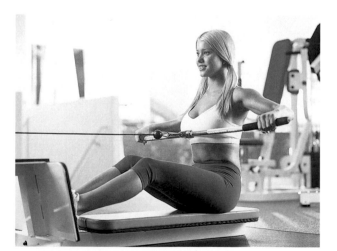

Seated Wide-Grip Cable Row

With your knees slightly bent and feet flat on the platform, sit erect with your abs tight and chest high. Take a wide overhand grip on the bar, arms extended. Keeping your shoulders down, pull the bar into your waist using your back muscles. Arch your back and bring your elbows behind you as far as you can. Squeeze your shoulder blades together and pause, then release, resisting the pull of the cable as you return to the start position. Don't lean forward or round your back on the return.

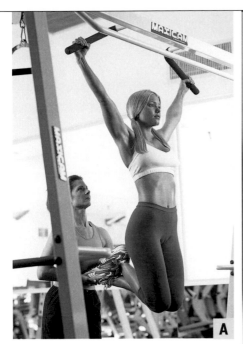

A

Assisted Wide-Grip Pull-Up

Pull-ups are truly one of the most basic exercises and a great way to build upper-body strength. Take a wide overhand grip on a pull-up bar and hang with your knees bent and ankles crossed behind you. Have a spotter place her hands under your ankles or the tops of your feet. Pull your body up by contracting your lats. Arch up as much as possible, aiming your sternum at the bar. Try to clear the bar with your chin, then return to the start position slowly and under control. Keep body swing to a minimum.

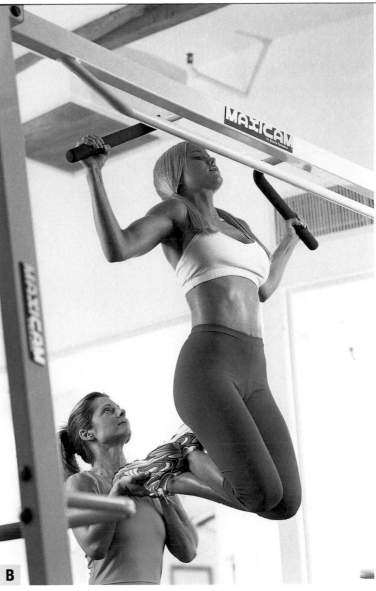

B

>>tip

Make a point of feeling the stretch at the beginning of each rep, as well as squeezing the peak contraction as hard as you can at the end of the range of motion. Anything less is cheating!

Basic Back Routine

Exercise	Sets	Reps
Assisted Wide-Grip Pull-Up	3–4	12–15
Seated Wide-Grip Cable Row	3–4	12–15
One-Arm Dumbbell Row	3–4	12–15*
*each side		

GETTING STARTED | Because the back is a large bodypart, you need to perform a variety of exercises to develop it fully. Don't neglect your lower back — it's the antagonist muscle to your abs, and it needs to be strong in order to support your abdominal workouts.

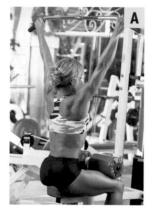
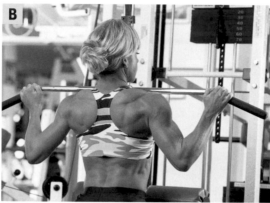

Lat Pulldown

After grasping the bar with your thumbs just outside the bends in the bar, sit erect on the seat and tuck your thighs under the pads. Using your hands as hooks to minimize using your arms to move the weight, pull the bar to the top of your chest while maintaining a slight arch in your lower back. Pause, then release under control and stretch.

Reverse-Grip Bent-Over Barbell Row

Stand erect with your feet close together, and bend your knees and hips about 45 degrees. Grasp the bar with an underhand (palms facing up) grip, hands about shoulder-width apart, and pull the bar toward your hips. Pause for a second at the top of the movement and squeeze your back. Keep your head up and abs tight, which helps to keep your back flat. On the return, try to push the bar away from your body for a stretch.

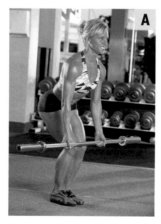
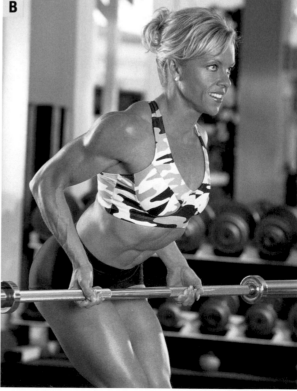

Standing One-Arm Dumbbell Row

Place your left hand on either a bench or the dumbbell rack for stability and grasp a dumbbell in your right hand. Get into a position similar to a lunge. Start with your arm extended toward the floor, then pull with your back to bring the weight up toward the side of your ribcage. At the top, squeeze your back before lowering the weight back to the start position, stretching your lat at the bottom.

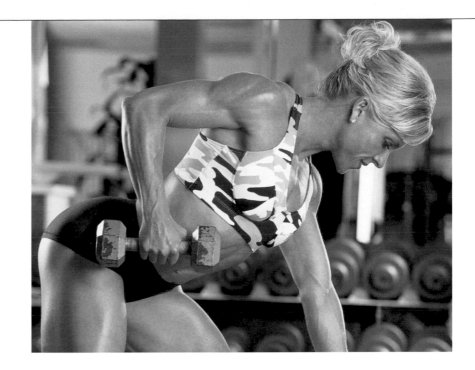

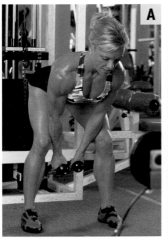 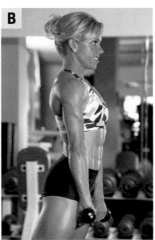

Cable Pull-Through (using rope)

This exercise is great for conditioning your lower back. To begin, hook a rope attachment to the low-pulley cable, then turn your back to it and reach between your legs to grasp the ends of the rope. Bend your knees slightly, and keep your back flat and your arms straight throughout the movement. Pull the weight up by pushing through your heels and pushing your hips forward, straightening your legs as you stand up. Don't use your shoulders or bend your arms. Bend your knees as you return to the start.

>>tip

Choose from exercises such as the bodyweight or weighted back extension, cable pull-through and deadlift to keep your lower back strong and injury-free.

Upper- & Lower-Back Routine

Exercise	Sets	Reps
Lat Pulldown	4	12
Reverse-Grip Bent-Over Barbell Row	3	20
Standing One-Arm Dumbbell Row	3	15*
Cable Pull-Through (using rope)	4	12

*each side

Seated Cable Row

Sitting with your knees bent and feet firmly planted, keep your abs tight and your chest high. Without rounding your back, lean forward slightly to grasp the cable attachment, then forcefully contract your back muscles to pull the handle toward your waist. Squeeze your shoulder blades together, hold for a moment and then release, resisting the pull of the weight as you return to the start position.

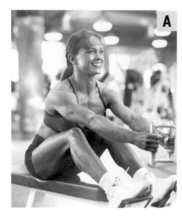
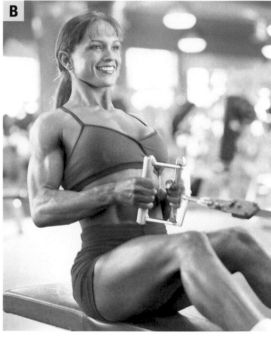

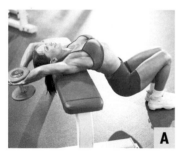
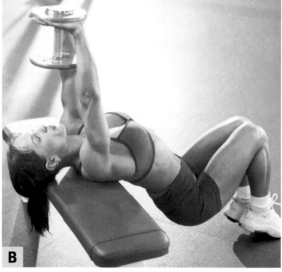

Dumbbell Pullover

Position yourself across a flat bench with your head and shoulder blades resting on it. Have a spotter hand you a dumbbell with your arms extended over your chest, palms flat against the inside edge of the weight. With your elbows bent slightly, lower the dumbbell under control behind your head. Keep your hips down to get that full stretch. Squeeze your lats to return to the start.

Machine Row

The Hammer Strength row machine can help build up the area that ties in your lower lats with the upper portion of your back. With your chest flush against the pad, reach straight out and grasp the handles with a neutral grip, then pull them toward your shoulders. Bring your elbows all the way back, getting a good contraction. Slowly release to the start position and feel the stretch through your lats.

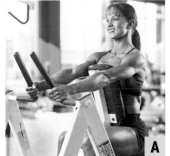 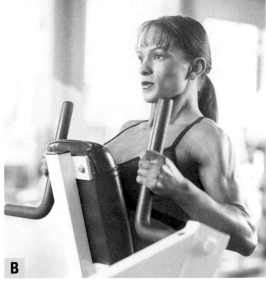

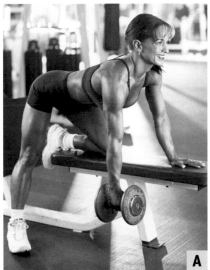 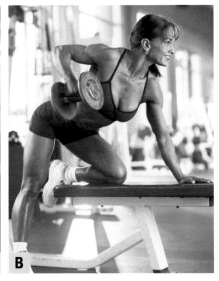

One-Arm Dumbbell Row

Position your left hand and shin on a flat bench, grasping a dumbbell in your right hand with your arm hanging straight down. Keeping your back flat and your arm close to your side, contract your back muscles while bending your elbow to pull the weight up to your side. Beware of turning your shoulder up in an effort to raise the weight; instead, try to keep your body square to the bench. After squeezing the muscle hard, return under control, going for a full stretch in the bottom position.

>>tip

Take your time — keep your rep speed slow to isolate your lats, low back or upper back. It may help to have a trainer or partner touch the target muscle as you perform an exercise.

Superset Back Routine

Exercise	Sets	Reps
Seated Cable Row —superset with—	2	10
Dumbbell Pullover	2	12
Machine Row —superset with—	2	15
One-Arm Dumbbell Row	2	12*

To perform a superset, do your reps for each exercise back-to-back with no rest in between.
*each side

GETTING STARTED | Back training can be hard enough without it being boring. Spice up your routine and enhance your development by modifying your grip widths and hand positions. Vary your workouts slightly each time to avoid muscular adaptation and stagnation.

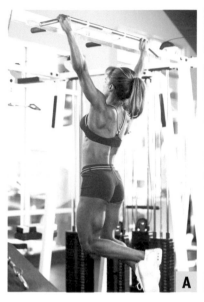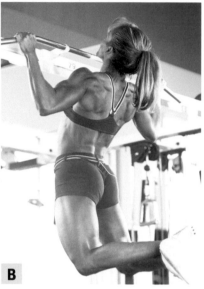

A B

Pull-Up

Grasp the bar with an overhand grip outside shoulder width, straighten your arms and let your body hang from the bar. Bend your knees and cross your ankles behind you. Slowly pull your body up until the top of your chest nearly touches the bar. As you move upward, focus on pulling your elbows down at an angle toward your ribcage, and keep your body straight without arching or swinging. Once your lats are completely contracted at the top, slowly return to the start position. Use a spotter if necessary.

Wide-Grip Lat Pulldown

Grasp the bar firmly with an overhand grip, your hands far outside shoulder width. Secure your legs under the kneepads, feet flat on the floor. Bend your elbows to pull the bar down to the top of your chest, arching your back slightly as you focus on keeping your elbows directly in line beneath the bar. Pause briefly with the bar right on top of your collarbone, then slowly return to the start position.

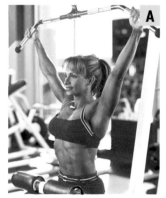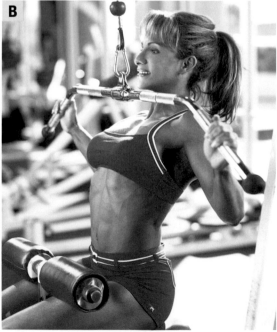

A B

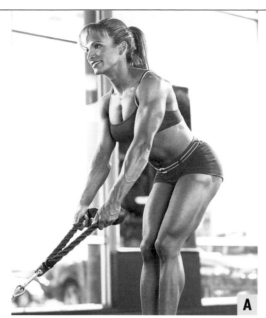

A

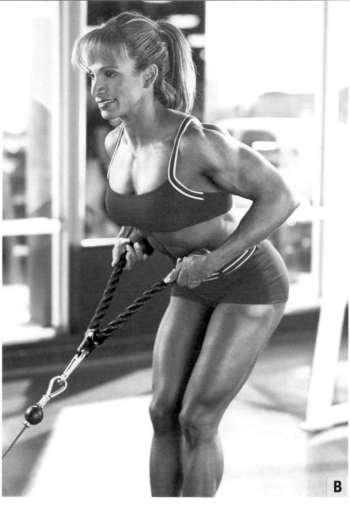

B

Bent-Over Cable Row (with rope)

Face a cable station and stand a few feet away from it with your feet together and knees bent slightly. Firmly grasp the ends of the rope attached to the low-pulley cable and lean forward from the hips so your torso is at a 45-degree angle. Keeping your abs contracted and your back flat, pull the ends of the rope to the sides of your waist by squeezing your shoulder blades together as you pull your elbows back. Extend your arms to return to the start.

>>tip

By giving both your chest and back equal attention in your training program, you can avoid creating a strength imbalance between these two bodyparts. If you train them on the same day, alternate which one you do first.

V-Taper Back Routine

Exercise	Sets	Reps
Pull-Up	3	10
Wide-Grip Lat Pulldown	3	12–15
Bent-Over Cable Row (with rope)	3	12–15
One-Arm Dumbbell Row	2	12*

*each side

GETTING STARTED | Aside from improving the way you look and feel, training your upper-back muscles may help prevent problems such as shoulder impingement and neck strain commonly caused by hunching over a computer keyboard or steering wheel every day.

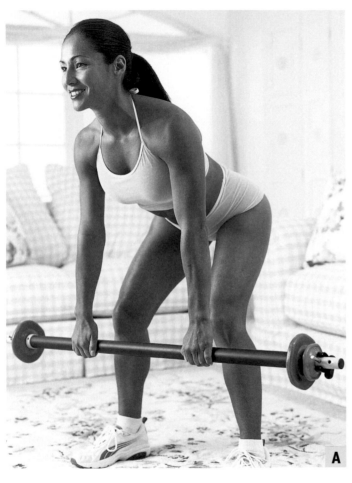

Bent-Over Barbell Row

Stand with your feet about shoulder-width apart with a slight bend in your knees. Bend forward at your hips about 45 degrees while keeping a slight arch in your lower back. Grasp the bar with a shoulder-width grip straight down in front of your legs, squeeze your shoulder blades together and pull the bar into your midsection, keeping your elbows close to your body. Pause, then control the return.

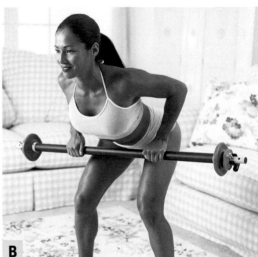

A   B

At-Home Back Routine

Exercise	Sets	Reps
Bent-Over Barbell Row	3–4	12–15
Dumbbell Pullover	3–4	12–15
One-Arm Dumbbell Row	3–4	12–15*
*each side		

>>tip

Keeping your neck and spine in proper alignment when you train with weights is crucial for injury prevention. In addition to making the exercises safer, they're also more effective.

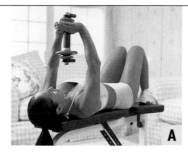

A

Dumbbell Pullover

Lie faceup on a flat bench and grasp a dumbbell with both hands, palms cupping the inside of the weight plate, arms extended over your chest. Keep your elbows bent slightly throughout the movement. Hinge at the shoulders to slowly lower the weight overhead until you feel a good stretch. Squeeze through your chest to return to the start.

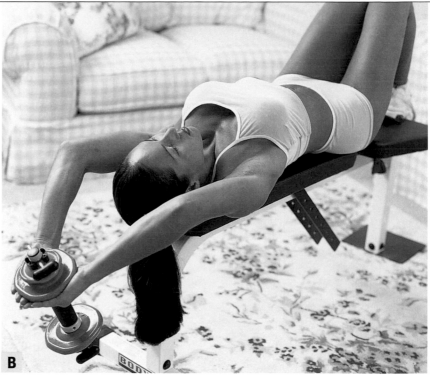

B

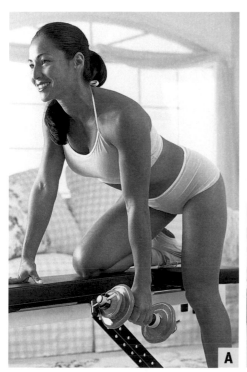

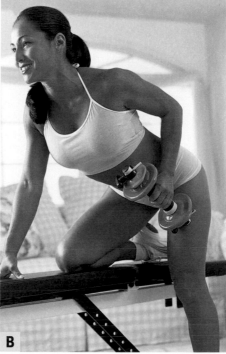

A   B

One-Arm Dumbbell Row

Rest your right hand and shin on a flat bench for support, keeping a slight arch in your lower back. Grasp a dumbbell in your left hand, arm extended, then squeeze your left shoulder blade toward the middle of your back and pull the weight close to your hip, keeping your elbow tight to your side. Repeat for reps, then switch sides. Keeping your torso inclined slightly changes the area of emphasis.

GETTING STARTED | Having a well-defined back isn't just about looking good — it's key to staying strong and injury-free. Not only does a fit back support the entire body, but it means better posture and less strain on other bodyparts such as your hips, knees and feet.

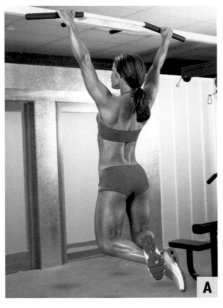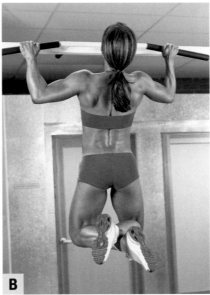

A B

Pull-Up

Start with an overhand grip (palms facing away) on the bar, slightly wider than shoulder width. Squeeze your shoulder blades together, arch your back, focus on your lats and pull your body up, aiming your chest toward the bar. Be aware that assistive machines allow you to use momentum and can create some bad habits. If you use an assistive machine, concentrate on keeping your back arched so that you develop ideal form.

One-Arm Dumbbell Row

With a dumbbell in your right hand, palm facing in, place your left knee and hand on a flat bench for support. Start with your abs tight, your back flat and slightly arched, and your head in a neutral position, looking at a point on the floor in front of you. With your right arm hanging down toward the floor, start the row by squeezing your shoulder blade and bending your elbow to bring the dumbbell up to your ribs, keeping your arm close to your side. Slowly lower to a full stretch. Repeat for reps, then switch sides.

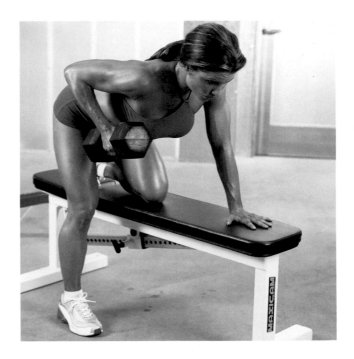

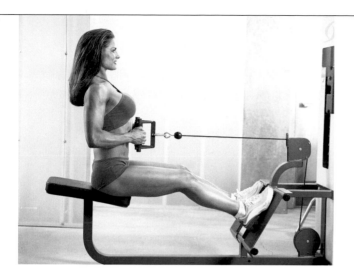

Seated Cable Row

Grasp the neutral V-grip handle with both hands and sit on the bench, feet flat on the platform. Keep your knees slightly bent, torso upright, abs tight and back slightly arched. Pull the handle toward your waist, keeping your arms close to the sides of your body. Bring your elbows as far back as possible and squeeze your shoulder blades together at the end of the movement. The rowing motion should come from your upper back, not your arms or lower back. Slowly extend your arms to return to the start, keeping your back erect.

Lat Pulldown

Start by taking an overhand grip on the pulldown bar, slightly wider than shoulder width. Sit down and position your thighs under the pads, feet flat on the floor. Keep your back slightly arched and squeeze your shoulder blades together as you pull the bar down to your upper chest. Pause and return under control to the start position.

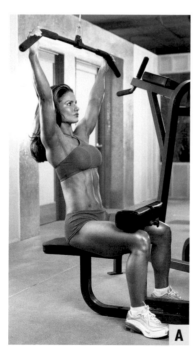
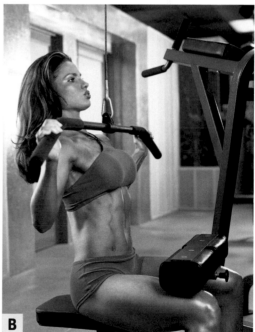

A B

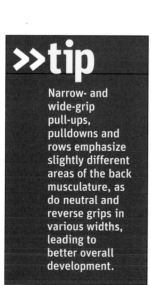

>>tip

Narrow- and wide-grip pull-ups, pulldowns and rows emphasize slightly different areas of the back musculature, as do neutral and reverse grips in various widths, leading to better overall development.

Heavy-Weight Back Routine

Exercise	Sets	Reps
Pull-Up	3–4	8–12
One-Arm Dumbbell Row	3–4	8–12*
Seated Cable Row	3–4	8–12
Lat Pulldown	3–4	8–12

*each side

Perfect Posture Routine

This program comprises six exercises. The first exercise of the workout will warm up the entire back musculature. The next five moves target specific areas by alternating between exercises that focus on the upper- and lower-back muscles. Rest two minutes between exercises and 1–2 minutes between sets. If you want to continue this program after four weeks but wish to build strength rather than muscle, increase the weights while decreasing the reps to 5–7 and the sets to two or three.

Exercise	WEEKS 1 & 2		WEEKS 3 & 4	
	Sets	Reps	Sets	Reps
Stiff-Legged Deadlift	3	8–12	4	8–12
Lat Pulldown	3	8–12	4	8–12
Back Extension	3	8–12	4	8–12
Inverted Row	3	8–12	4	8–12
Reverse Back Extension	3	8–12	4	8–12
One-Arm Dumbbell Row	3	8–12*	4	8–12*

*each side

Beginner's Back Routine

This is a progressive six-week program using moderate weight. Do the exercises listed twice a week, resting 45–60 seconds between sets.

WEEKS 1 & 2 Exercise	Sets	Reps
Assisted Pull-Up	1–2	12–15
Machine Row	1–2	8–12

WEEKS 3 & 4 Exercise	Sets	Reps
Lat Pulldown	2	10–12
One-Arm Dumbbell Row	2	10–12*

WEEKS 5 & 6 Exercise	Sets	Reps
Assisted Pull-Up	1–2	12–15
Lat Pulldown	2	8–12
One-Arm Dumbbell Row	2	10–12*

*each side

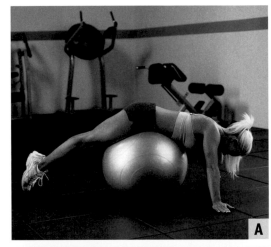

A

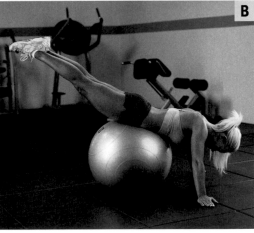

B

Reverse Back Extension

Lie facedown on an exercise ball, legs extended straight behind you with your toes touching the floor. Place your hands on the floor in front of you for stability. Squeeze through your low back to raise both legs evenly as high as possible, then slowly lower and repeat.

Advanced Back Routine

This program splits your back training into two days. After the first workout, avoid training your back for 48 hours to give it enough rest. Rest for 45–60 seconds between sets.

WORKOUT 1 Exercise	Sets	Reps
Pull-Up	2–3	10–12
Lat Pulldown	2–3	10–12
Seated Cable Row	2–3	8–12
Bent-Over Barbell Row	2–3	10–15

WORKOUT 2 Exercise	Sets	Reps
Standing Lat Pulldown	2–3	10–12
Inverted Row	2	8–12
One-Arm Dumbbell Row	2	8–12*
*each side		

At-Home Back Routine

All you need is a flat bench, a barbell and a pair of adjustable dumbbells, or multiple dumbbells of multiple weights. Beginners should do lighter sets of 12–15 reps.

Exercise	Sets	Reps
Bent-Over Barbell Row	5	15, 12, 10, 8, 24
One-Arm Dumbbell Row	4	8–12*
Bent-Over Dumbbell Row	4	10, 15, 25, 30
*each side		

Standing Lat Pulldown
(not shown)

Stand erect behind the seat at the lat pulldown station, grasping the bar just outside shoulder width. Squeeze your lats to pull the bar down to your thighs, keeping your arms extended. Return under control.

Inverted Row

Lie faceup on the floor under an Olympic bar placed just beyond arm's reach in a squat rack or Smith machine. Align yourself so the bar is above your chest, then grasp it with a slightly wider than shoulder-width overhand grip. Using the power of only your back muscles, pull your upper body to the bar so your chest touches it. Keep your body completely flat throughout the motion. Pause, lower and repeat.

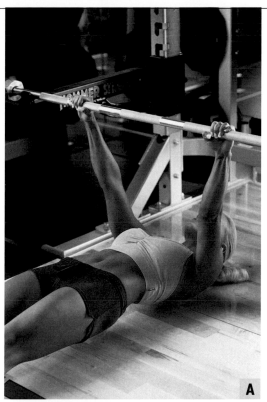

A

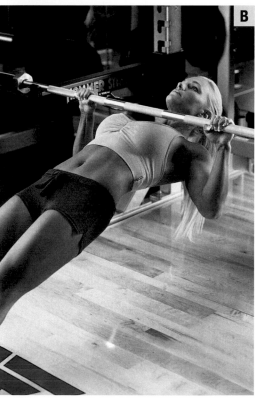

B

legs

Chapter SIX

Long, Lean Legs

Everyone wants a shapely lower half with sleek curves in all the right places. But our legs should be more than just visually appealing — they need to be strong enough to take us wherever we'd like to go. From top to bottom, muscular balance is key.

GETTING STARTED | Most women gain weight and store bodyfat easily in the hips and thighs, making these areas challenging to firm and shape. To boost your own bottom line, focus on compound, multijoint leg exercises. Your glutes could become one of your best assets!

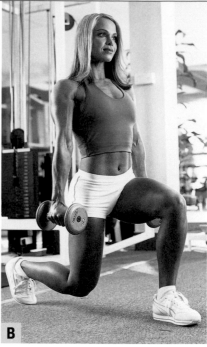

Walking Lunge

Stand erect holding a pair of dumbbells or put your hands on your hips. Take a long step forward with one leg and lift up onto the ball of your back foot. Keeping your chest high and shoulders back, bend your knees to drop your hips straight down until your front thigh is parallel to the floor. Don't let your back knee touch the floor or your forward knee move past your toes. Press back up through your front leg as you bring your back foot forward, then take another large step forward with the opposite leg. Keep the movement smooth and continuous.

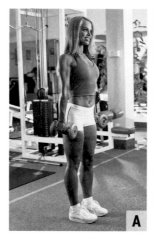

A B

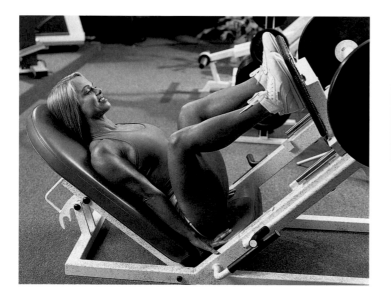

Leg Press

Sit in a leg-press machine, placing your feet high and slightly wider than shoulder-width apart on the platform. Keeping your back and hips flat against the pads, lower the sled until your knees form 90-degree angles. Pause briefly, then press back up to the starting position until your legs are straight but not locked. Focus on pressing through your heels for more glute emphasis. Don't lower the sled too far, which forces your lower back to lift off the backpad.

Leg & Glute Routine

Exercise	Sets	Reps
Walking Lunge	2–3	12–15*
Leg Press	2–3	12–15
Romanian Deadlift	2–3	12–15

*each side

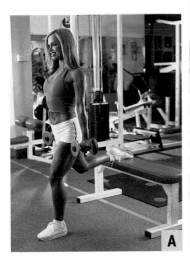

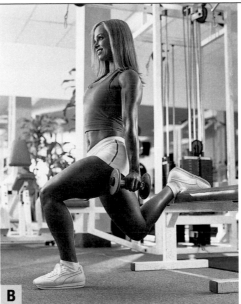

A **B**

Single-Leg Squat

Stand erect 3–4 feet in front of either an exercise ball (more challenging) or a flat bench placed behind you. Extend one leg back and place that foot on top of the bench/ball. With your hands on your hips or holding dumbbells, lower your hips by bending both knees until your front thigh is parallel to the floor. Don't allow your front knee to move past your toes. Focusing on your glutes, press back up through your front foot to the starting position and repeat for reps, then switch legs.

Step-Up With Knee Lift

Facing an 8–10-inch-high step or box, put your hands on your hips or grasp a pair of dumbbells. Place your right foot on top of the step. Lifting your body by pressing through your right foot, step up and kick your left knee upward until your left thigh is parallel to the floor. Return your left foot to the floor, leaving your right foot on the step. Be sure not to bounce off the floor when you step down. Repeat for reps, then switch legs.

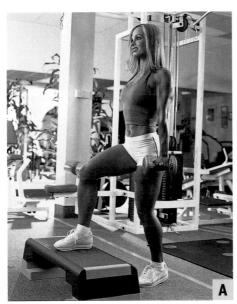

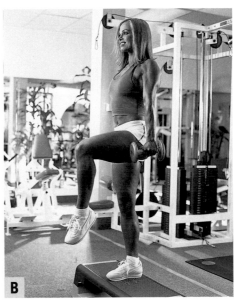

A **B**

Leg & Glute Routine

Exercise	Sets	Reps
Single-Leg Squat	2–3	12–15*
Step-Up With Knee Lift	2–3	12–15*
Exercise-Ball Lying Bridge	2–3	12–15

*each side

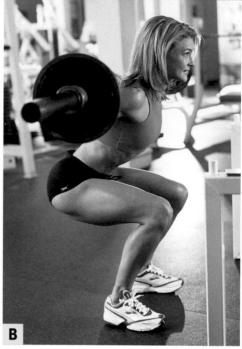

Back Squat

Stand erect in a squat rack (not shown) with your feet hip-width apart, toes pointed slightly outward, a loaded bar across your traps and hands spaced wide to stabilize the bar. Facing straight ahead, drop into the squat by bending your knees and moving your hips back, keeping your chin and chest up. Descend to the point where your thighs are parallel to the floor, then drive through your heels to reverse the motion and return to the start position.

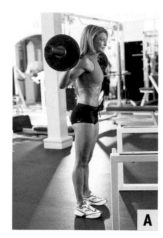

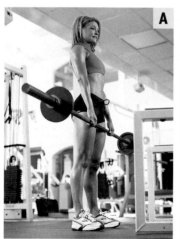

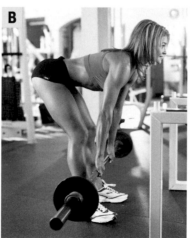

Romanian Deadlift

Stand behind a loaded barbell placed on a rack at hip height. Grasp the bar with an overhand or staggered grip and step back from the rack. Stand erect with your chest high, back slightly arched and knees slightly bent, feet hip-width apart. As you lean forward from your hips, slide the bar down your legs, maintaining the arch in your lower back. Reverse the motion as you push your hips forward. Come all the way back up to the start position and squeeze your glutes.

Superset Leg Routine

Exercise	Sets	Reps
Back Squat —superset with—	3	10–12
Jump Squat	3	20
Romanian Deadlift —superset with—	3	10–12
Reverse Lunge	3	20*

*each side
Do each of the paired exercises back-to-back with no rest in between.

>>tip

Before training legs, warm up on a stationary bike, treadmill or elliptical trainer for 10 minutes to increase flexibility and help prevent injury.

Jump Squat

Stand erect in front of a mirror with your feet hip-width apart, knees slightly bent (A). Squat down — hips back, head and chest up (B) — then explode upward, propelling yourself off the floor and reaching as high as you can with your hands (C). When you land, descend into the squat position as your arms swing back behind you and repeat immediately.

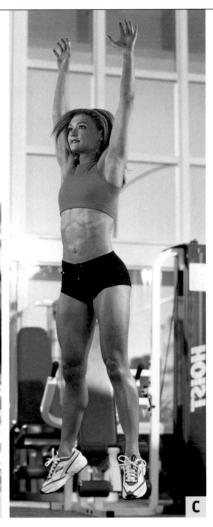

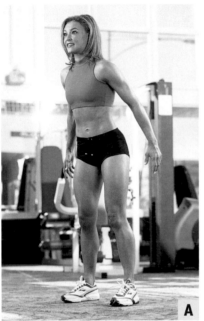

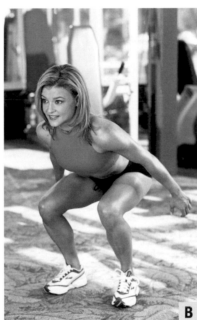

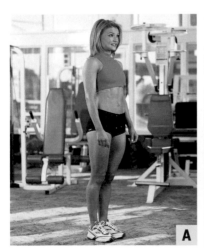

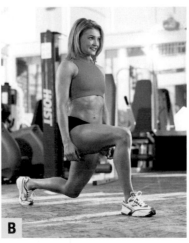

Reverse Lunge

Stand erect in front of a mirror, chest up, shoulders back, hands down by your sides. Take a giant step backward with your left foot and drop your hips toward the floor so your front knee forms a 90-degree angle. Reverse the motion and press back up by driving through your right foot, returning your left foot to the starting position. Alternate sides for reps.

GETTING STARTED | Squats, lunges, leg presses. Odds are, you already do these fundamental leg exercises. But to really sculpt and define your thighs, you must advance your training. This unilateral-heavy routine will strengthen your core and stabilizing muscles.

Cable Step-Up

Attach a D-handle to a low-pulley cable. Place a flat bench in front of you and stand facing away from the cable station. Grasp the handle with your right hand in front of your shoulder and place your right foot atop the bench. Push through your right foot to stand on top of the bench; squeeze your right glute and pause at the top. Slowly lower back down by bending your right knee, making sure it doesn't go beyond your toes. Repeat for reps, then switch sides. Don't bounce off the floor with your nonworking leg.

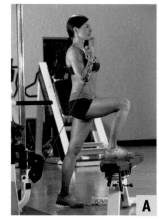
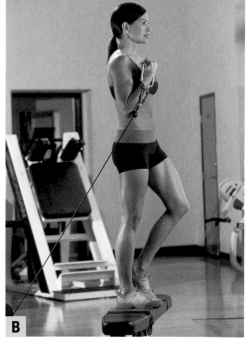

A B

Standing Leg Extension & Hip Flexion

With your back to the weight stack of a cable station, stand erect just to the left of it and hook your right foot inside a D-handle attached to the low-pulley cable so you have a direct line of pull. Keep your left knee slightly bent and your hands on your hips or grasping a handle for balance. With your right leg bent about 45 degrees at the hip, bend your knee about 90 degrees with your foot flexed (A). Fully extend your right leg (B), then return to the start and repeat for reps. Next, keep your knee bent and lift your thigh until it's parallel to the floor (C), then return to 45 degrees; repeat for reps. Switch legs and repeat the sequence of moves.

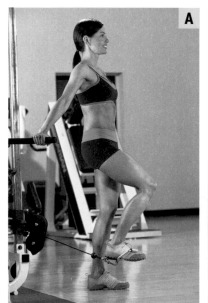
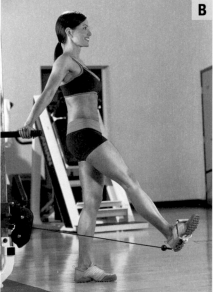
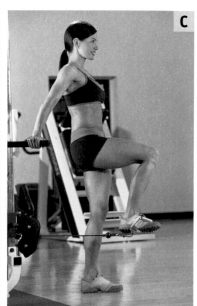

A B C

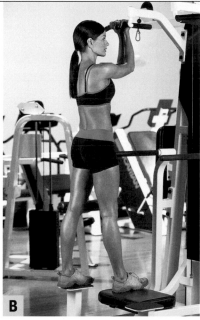

A **B**

Standing Leg Press

Stand erect at an assisted pull-up/ dip machine with your left foot on the left step and your right foot on the middle of the assist platform. Place both hands on your hips or lightly grasp the handle for balance. Push down on the platform through your heel until your right leg is fully extended. Resist the platform's return until your thigh is past parallel to the floor. Repeat for reps, then switch sides.

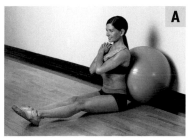

A **B**

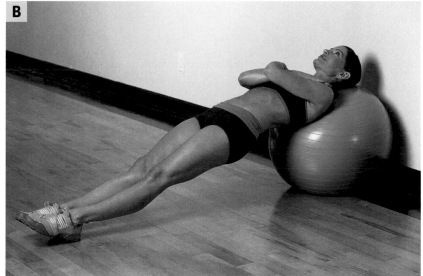

Seated Exercise-Ball Bridge

Place an exercise ball against a wall and sit snugly against it so your body forms a 90-degree angle at the hips, legs extended in front of you. Your shoulders should be higher than the top of the ball. Dig your heels into the floor and extend your hips to lift your pelvis, creating a straight line with your body. Keeping your core tight, squeeze your glutes and shoulder blades for 1–2 seconds. Lower your glutes to the floor and repeat for reps.

Stabilizing-Strength Routine

Exercise	Sets	Reps
Cable Step-Up	3	12–15*
Standing Leg Extension & Hip Flexion	3	15*
Standing Leg Press	3	15*
Seated Exercise-Ball Bridge	3	20

*each side

GETTING STARTED | Wouldn't you love to change your thighs? Running, cycling and kick-boxing are great ways to burn calories and fat, but they won't give you shapely legs on their own. You need some targeted leg training, and you can even do it at home in limited time.

Plié Squat

Begin with your feet spaced wide, toes pointing out slightly. With your head up and back straight, hold a dumbbell by one end with both hands between your legs. Lower into a sitting position or until your thighs are roughly parallel to the floor. Keeping your weight on your heels, press through your feet and push your hips forward to return to the starting position.

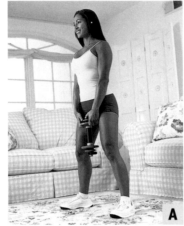

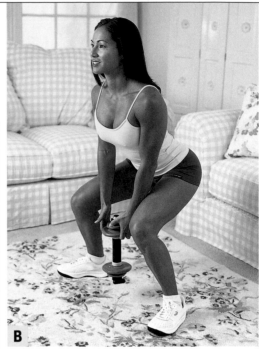

A **B**

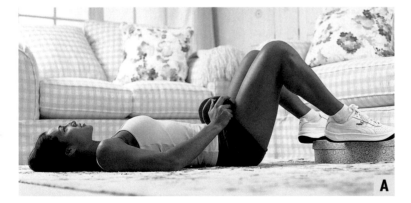

A

B

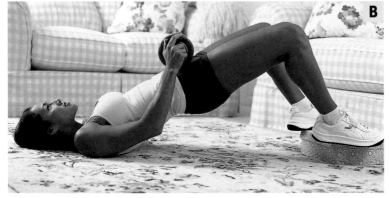

Hip Raise

Lie faceup on the floor with both knees bent and your feet up on a slightly elevated platform (such as an aerobic step or phone book) just beyond hip-width apart. Place a dumbbell across your lower abs and slowly lift your hips toward the ceiling, pushing your knees out and away from your body. You'll feel your bodyweight on your shoulder blades and the balls of your feet. Squeeze your glutes and hold for a moment, then slowly lower.

>>tip

When deciding your order of exercises, remember this rule: Go from largest muscles to smallest. For legs, then, target your quads, hams and glutes before your abductors, adductors and calves.

Front Lunge

Stand erect with your feet hip-width apart, holding dumbbells at your sides. Take a large step forward with one leg, bending your front knee to a 90-degree angle with your thigh parallel to the floor. Your back knee should almost touch down. With your weight on your front heel, contract your quad, hamstrings and glutes to push back up to the starting position. Alternate sides for reps.

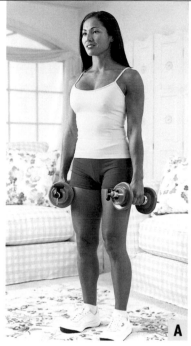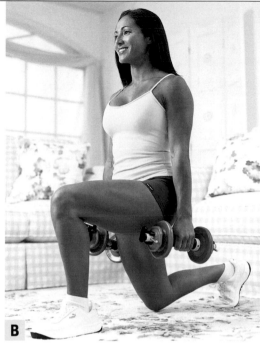

Calf Raise

Stand erect with your feet hip-width apart, grasping a chair or wall for balance. Slowly raise your heels until you're on tiptoe, balancing your bodyweight on the balls of your feet. Pause, then lower. (For a greater range of motion, stand on a step where you can fully lower your heels.)

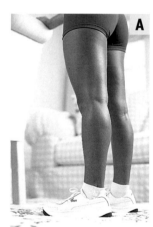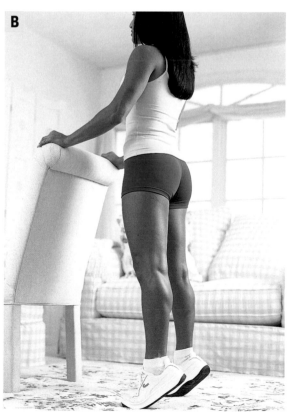

At-Home Leg Routine

Exercise	Sets	Reps
Plié Squat	3–4	15–20
—superset with—		
Hip Raise	3–4	15–20
Front Lunge	3–4	15–20*
—superset with—		
Calf Raise	3–4	15–20

*each side
Beginners should start with one superset each, doing each of the paired exercises back-to-back with no rest in between.

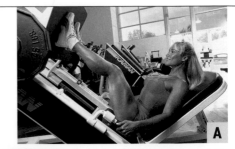

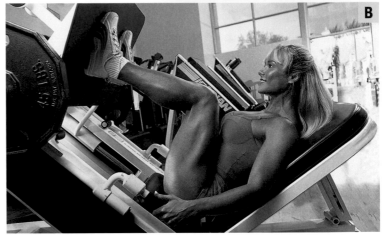

Leg Press

With your back and hips fully supported by the pads, place your feet shoulder-width apart in the center of the platform. Slowly lower the sled so your knees approach your chest, making sure your glutes don't lift up off the pad, which increases the risk of injury. At the bottom, keep your heels pressed firmly against the platform and forcefully drive the weight up under control, stopping short of locking out your knees.

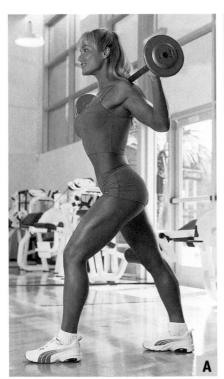

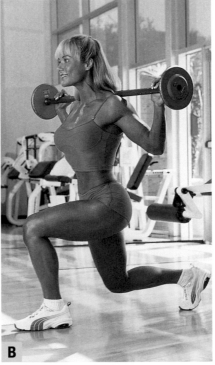

Stationary Barbell Lunge

Standing erect with a barbell positioned across the back of your shoulders, take a step forward and firmly plant your foot in the start position. Keeping your chest lifted and feet facing forward, lower your body until your back knee nearly touches the floor, being careful not to let your front knee extend past your toes. Press back up through both thighs, and repeat for reps using a steady, rhythmic pace before switching legs. Stay in place with both feet on the floor.

Leg Extension

Sit in the machine, adjusting the backpad so your knees are just beyond the edge of the seat and your back and thighs are flush against the pads. Push the ankle pad all the way up by extending your legs, squeeze your quads as hard as you can without locking your knees and return slowly, resisting the weight. Stop short of allowing the plates to rest on the stack to keep tension on the muscles. You could do this exercise with your toes pointing in, as shown, to put slightly more emphasis on the outer part of your quads.

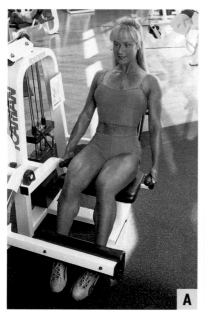

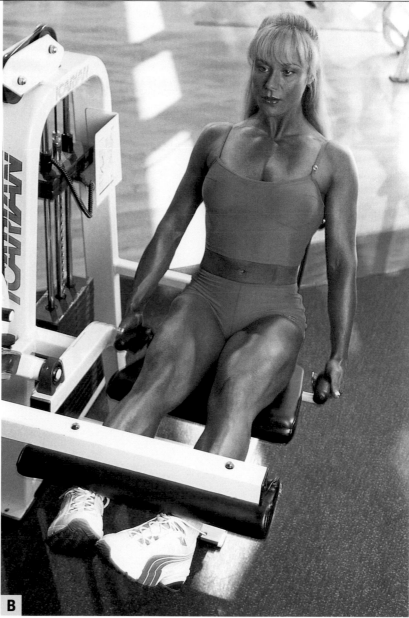

A   B

>>tip

If you're having trouble losing fat, train your legs hard once a week and try plyometrics or sprint training on another day on top of your usual cardio workouts.

Quad-Focused Routine

Exercise	Sets	Reps
Leg Press or Squat	3–4	10–15
Stationary Barbell Lunge	3	10–12*
Leg Extension	3–4	10–15
*each side		

Weighted Step-Up

Standing erect with dumbbells at your sides, plant one foot on top of a bench. Push through the heel of that foot to lift your body, squeezing through your glutes, until you're standing erect atop the bench. Reverse the movement under control to return to the start position, touching your back foot to the floor only briefly. Repeat for reps, then switch legs.

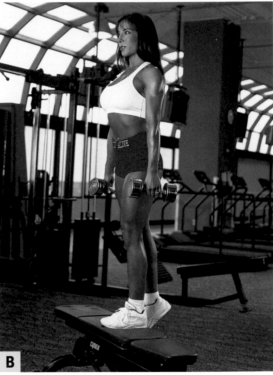

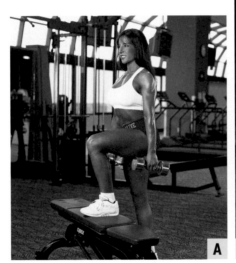

A   B

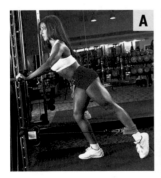

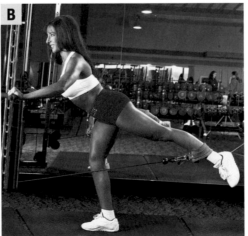

A   B

Cable Hip Extension

Strap on an ankle cuff attached to a low-pulley cable and stand facing the weight stack, hips square to the machine and torso inclined slightly. Bending your base leg for support, turn out the toe of your cuffed foot slightly to hit the abductors (outer thigh) a bit more. Push that leg straight up and back, keeping it as tight and straight as possible to hit your glutes. Squeeze at the top, then return slowly under control. Don't let your foot touch the floor. Use a steady, even tempo, repeating for reps before switching legs.

Dumbbell Hip Extension

Kneel at the end of a flat bench, then lean forward so your torso is supported by the bench and your legs hang off. Bend your knees and bring your heels together, toes and knees out and away from your body. Start with no weight until you get used to the movement. Later you can add light ankle weights or a light dumbbell. Lift your legs as you press your heels toward the ceiling, squeezing your glutes as tightly as possible. Go just high enough to feel the contraction through your glutes — it's actually a small movement — then return under control to the start position. Those with low-back problems can perform the exercise on the floor.

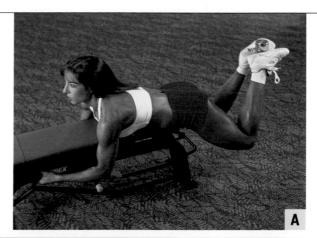

A

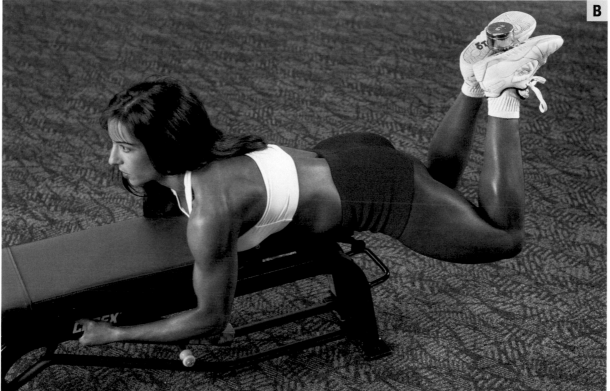

B

>>**tip**

For glute-focused cardio training, choose the stair-stepper, walk or jog uphill, or use the treadmill set at an incline. Every time you work your glutes, you want to feel it!

Glute-Focused Routine

Exercise	Sets	Reps
Weighted Step-Up	1	25 (no weight)*
	4	15–20*
Cable Hip Extension	3	20–25*
Dumbbell Hip Extension	4	25–30

*each side

GETTING STARTED | If leaner glutes and thighs are your top priorities, do two leg workouts a week, using high reps and less resistance. This routine targets each muscle group within the thighs and glutes. Start with heavier weight and decrease it as the reps increase.

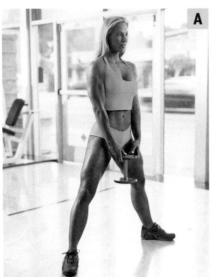 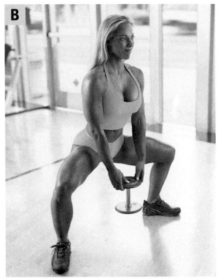

Plié Squat

Place your feet fairly wide with your toes turned out about 45 degrees. Stand erect with your shoulders up and back and your chest out, holding a dumbbell by one end with both hands between your legs. Descend until your knees form 90-degree angles, making sure they go directly over your toes, then press up through your heels while squeezing your glutes and hams. Rise about three-quarters of the way to where your knees are slightly bent.

Smith-Machine Reverse Lunge

Stand under the bar with your feet together, unrack the bar and position it comfortably across the back of your shoulders, then step forward with both feet. Keep your torso erect and your abs tight. Take a big step back with one foot and descend so your front knee forms a 90-degree angle, keeping your forward knee above your foot. To return to the start, step forward with your back foot while pressing through the heel of your front foot. Go right back down into the lunge position using a moderate pace. Do all reps for one side, then switch legs.

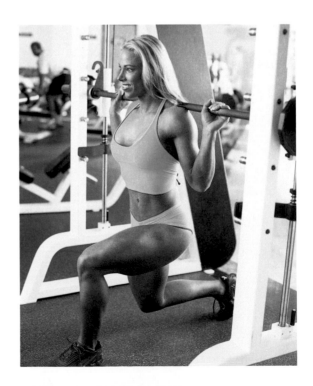

>>tip

Alternate phases in which you lift a bit heavier with lower-weight phases in which you use higher reps. This helps you avoid a plateau, keeps things interesting and can prevent injuries resulting from overuse.

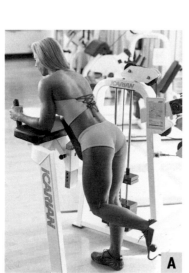
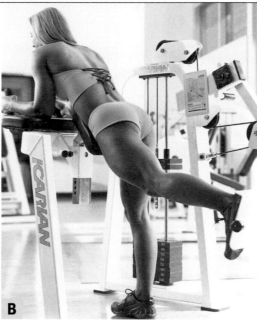

Standing Butt Blaster

Stand in the machine with your hips and shoulders square, forearms on the pad and left foot against the platform. Extend your working leg back, pushing through your entire foot and squeezing your glutes hard at the top of the movement. Control the negative as you allow the platform to return only part of the way to prevent the weight stack from touching. Starting with your knee at a 90-degree angle keeps tension on the glutes. Don't go too fast or you'll end up using momentum.

A   B

Leg Extension

Sit with your back flush against the pad and feet under the ankle pad. With your feet flexed toward the ceiling, squeeze your quads to straighten your legs against the resistance. Pause at the top, squeeze and release slowly so your legs return nearly to the start position. Don't let the stack touch down to keep tension on your quads.

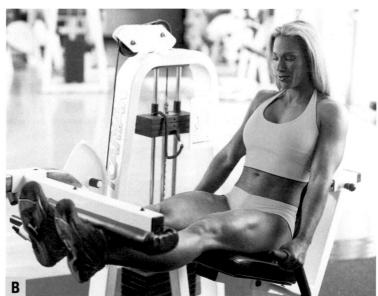

B

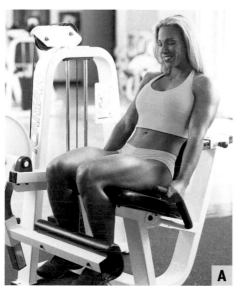

A

High-Rep Leg & Glute Routine

Exercise	Sets	Reps
Plié Squat	3	20, 30, 40
Smith-Machine Reverse Lunge	3	15, 20, 25*
Standing Butt Blaster	3	30, 40, 50*
Leg Extension	3	30, 30, 30

*each side

GETTING STARTED | Rather than isolating individual muscles of the legs, the compound exercises described here work the multiple quadriceps, hamstrings and gluteal muscles simultaneously. Use a full range of motion to boost the effectiveness.

Back Squat

Standing erect, take a wider-than-shoulder-width grip on an Olympic bar positioned just below shoulder height in a squat rack. Center it behind your head, resting it across your traps and rear delts, and lift it off the rack. With your feet shoulder-width apart and toes pointed out slightly, lower your hips and bend your knees until your thighs are about parallel to the floor. Don't allow your knees to move beyond your toes. Reverse direction by extending your knees and pushing your hips forward.

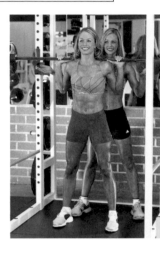
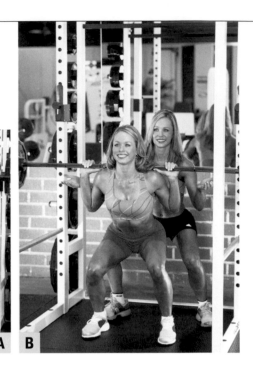

A B

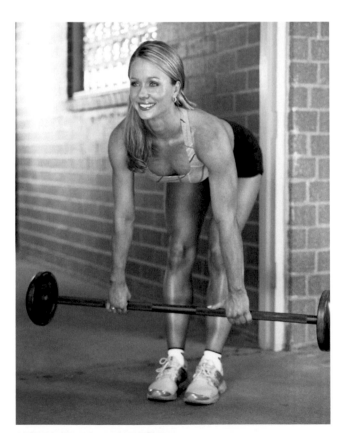

Stiff-Legged Deadlift

Stand erect with your feet roughly hip-width apart with a straight bar or dumbbells in your hands, arms extended. Lean forward at the hips, keeping your knees just slightly bent, back arched and eyes forward. Lower the bar to about mid-shin level, then contract your hamstrings and glutes as you straighten from your hips. Keep the bar close to your legs as you rise. Try to use primarily your hamstrings and glutes, not your lower back. As you return to the start, extend just slightly beyond upright to get the fullest contraction possible.

>>tip

A barbell can be difficult to control, so beginners should use a broomstick or very lightweight Body Bar until you master the technique and feel comfortable doing these exercises.

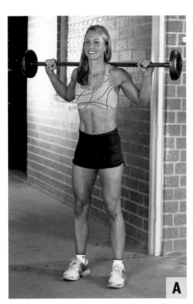
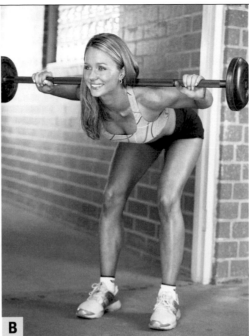

A **B**

Good Morning

Begin as you would with the back squat, except use a short straight bar or an EZ-bar to lessen the load. Standing erect, position the bar atop your traps and keep a slight bend in your knees. Arch your back and bend forward at the hips until your back is parallel to the floor, keeping your eyes up and midsection tight. Squeeze your hams and glutes to reverse the movement and return to the start.

Front Squat

Position an Olympic bar across your front delts and hold your upper arms parallel to the floor, arms crossed and hands palms-down over the bar. Don't let your elbows drop and don't bend forward — the weight will roll forward and pull you off-balance. Standing erect, squat down as you would in the back squat, then press through your heels and extend your knees to return to the start. If you use dumbbells, place the flat part atop your front delts.

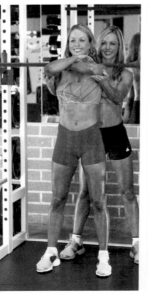
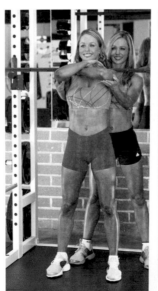
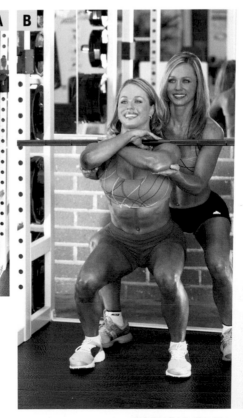

A **B**

Barbell Leg Routine

Exercise	Sets	Reps
Back Squat	3	12–15
Stiff-Legged Deadlift	3	12–15
Good Morning	3	12–15
Front Squat	3	12–15

GETTING STARTED | Our legs endure count-less hours of bending, squatting, cycling and walking, all courtesy of the knees. If you want to keep running, jumping and lifting, try this injury-prevention program. Many of the exercises also strengthen and define the thighs.

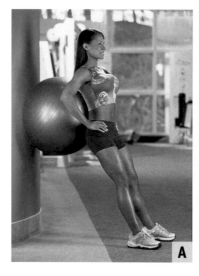
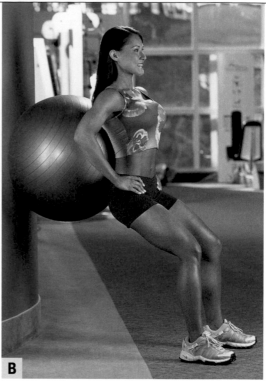

Exercise-Ball Squat

Place an exercise ball against a wall and stand erect with your low back firmly against it, feet out in front of you and shoulder-width apart. Bend your knees and roll the ball down the wall to move into a mini-squat position, about one-third of a full squat. Push through your heels to return to the top. As you gain strength, move into lower squat positions.

A B

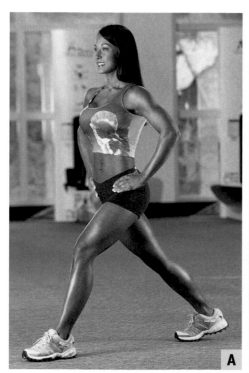
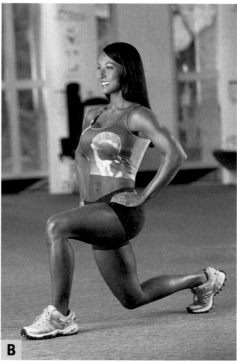

Reverse Lunge

This exercise places the entire weight of the body on one knee, so stand near and grasp a station-ary object if neces-sary. Standing erect, begin by taking a large step back with one foot, then bend your knees to lower your hips until your back knee almost touches the floor. Press back up through your front foot and bring your back foot forward. Repeat for reps, then switch sides.

A B

Horizontal Leg Press

Sit snugly in the machine and place your feet hip-width apart near the top of the platform to put more emphasis on your glutes. Release the safeties and slowly bend your knees to 90-degree angles, keeping your low back on the backpad. Push through your heels to return to the start under control. To target your quad muscles, place your feet near the bottom of the platform. In both positions, be careful not to let your knees move beyond your toes.

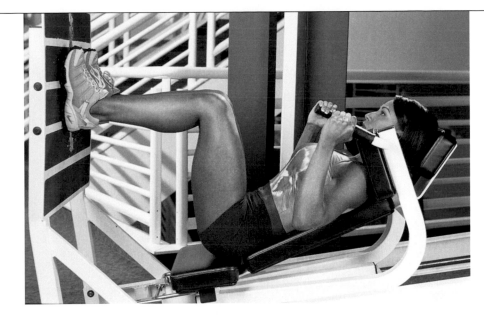

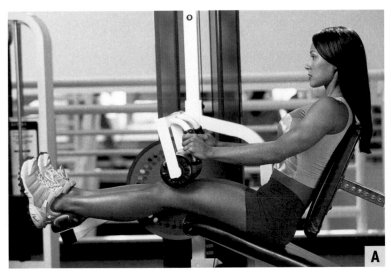

Seated Hamstring Curl

Sit snugly in the machine, placing the backs of your ankles on top of the pad. Contract your hams to press it down and back toward your body till your knees form 90-degree angles. Release slowly without hyperextending your knees at the top.

Healthy-Knees Routine

Exercise	Sets	Reps
Exercise-Ball Squat	3	10
Reverse Lunge	3	10*
Horizontal Leg Press	3	10
Seated Hamstring Curl	3	10

*each side

GETTING STARTED | Kick your leg routine up a notch by adding novel exercises. Lateral hops will help increase your functional capacity for sports and everyday activities, while dorsiflexion strengthens your anterior tibialis to prevent painful shinsplints.

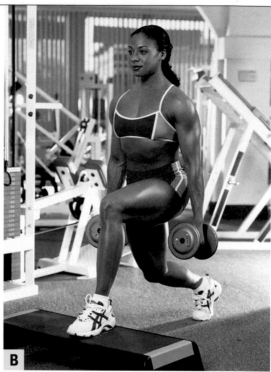

Split Squat

Stand erect holding a dumb-bell in each hand. Step 2–3 feet forward with your weaker leg onto a step or platform; this is the start position. Bend both knees and descend until your front thigh is parallel to the floor. Push through the heel of your front foot to return to the start position, keeping your chest up, eyes looking straight ahead and spine aligned throughout. Repeat for reps, then switch legs.

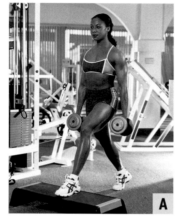

A   B

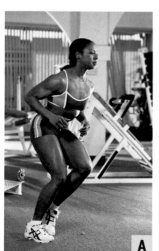

A

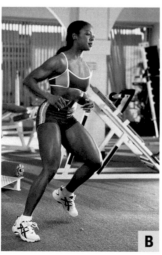

B

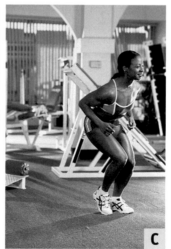

C

Lateral Hops

Place two markers 3 feet apart. Stand over one marker and get in an athletic stance — bend your elbows and knees, keep your abs tight and lean slightly forward (A). Jump sideways (B) from one marker to the other (C) and back for the allotted time, using your legs to absorb the impact and spending as little time as possible on the floor. Gradually increase the distance between markers.

Leg Routine

Exercise	Sets	Reps
Split Squat	3	12–15*
Lateral Hops	3	20–30 sec.
Lying Leg Curl	3	12–15
Dorsiflexion	3	12–15*

*each side

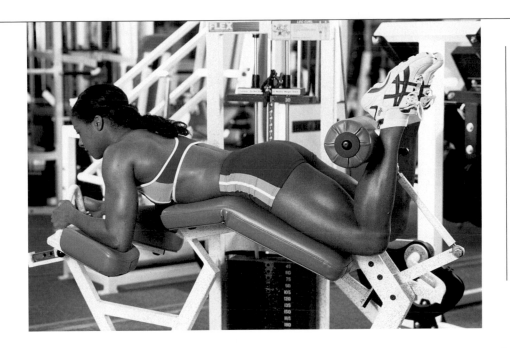

Lying Leg Curl

Lie facedown on the bench and place your heels under the ankle rollers. Grasp the handles, squeeze your shoulder blades together and raise your chest off the pad. Keeping your hips pressed into the pad, contract your hamstrings and bend your knees to raise the ankle rollers, bringing them as close to your glutes as possible. Lower to the start position without letting the weights touch the stack.

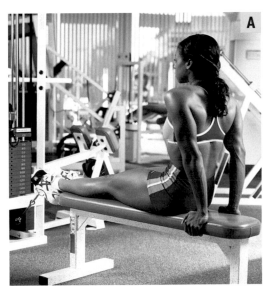

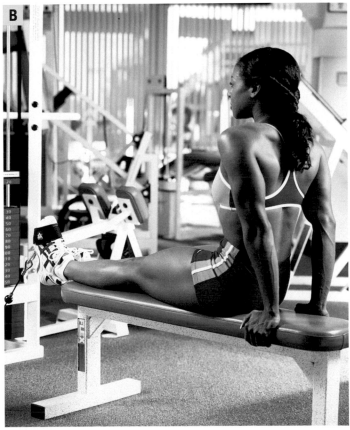

Dorsiflexion

Sit lengthwise on a bench placed perpendicular to a cable station so your feet and ankles hang over the edge closest to the weight stack. Grasp the sides of the bench near your glutes and have a spotter attach an ankle cuff connected to the low-pulley cable around the ball of one foot. Keeping your knees slightly bent, pull the toes of the cuffed foot as far as you can toward your shin. Repeat for reps, then switch legs.

Barbell Leg Routine

Exercise	Sets	Reps
Lunge Around the Clock	1–2	5–10*
Barbell Hack Squat	3	10–12
One-Leg Stiff-Legged Deadlift	3	10–12*

*each side

Lunge Around the Clock

Stand with your feet hip-width apart and rest a barbell across your traps, grasping it outside your shoulders. Pretend you're standing in the middle of a clock — 12:00 is straight ahead, 3:00 and 9:00 are straight out to the sides and 6:00 is straight behind you. Lunge forward with your right foot to the 12:00 position (A). Do a normal lunge, stopping when your right thigh is about parallel to the floor. Push back up to the start position. Lunge forward to the 2:00 position (B) with your toes pointed out slightly. Return to the start. Lunge far out to your side to the 3:00 position (C), keeping your foot pointing forward with your toes turned out slightly. As you lunge down, your left leg should be straight. Return to the start. Lunge back to the 5:00 position (D), lowering your hips until your left thigh is about parallel to the floor. Lunge straight back to the 6:00 position (E), as if doing a reverse lunge. Return to the start. This counts as one rep. Repeat the sequence with your left leg, going to the 12:00, 10:00, 9:00, 8:00 and 6:00 positions. Alternate right and left legs.

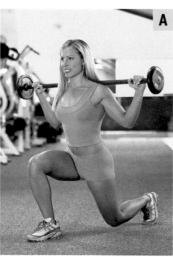
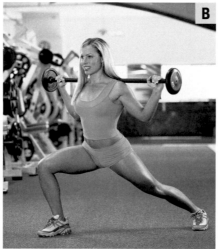
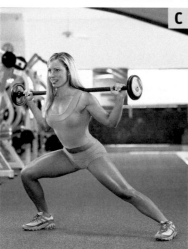
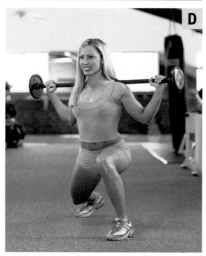
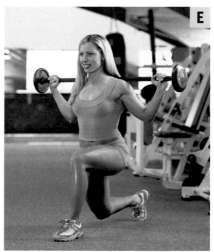

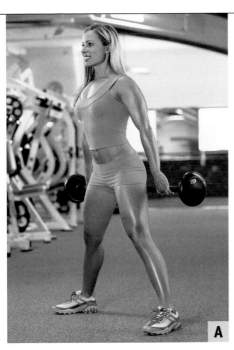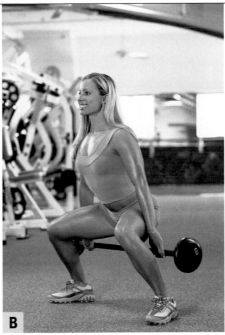

A **B**

Barbell Hack Squat

Stand with your feet at least 4 inches wider than shoulder width, turning your toes out slightly. Grasp a barbell with an overhand, shoulder-width grip behind you — the bar should be just below your glutes. Keep your abs tight, your back flat and your focus straight ahead as you lower your hips until your thighs are parallel to the floor. Hold for a moment, then return to the start by pushing through your heels.

One-Leg Stiff-Legged Deadlift

Stand erect with your feet close together and up on your left toes. Grasp a barbell with an overhand grip and extended arms. Bend your right knee slightly as you slowly lift your left leg straight back and up. Simultaneously hinge at the hips to lower your torso, keeping it in line with your left leg. Contract through your hams and glutes to push your hips forward and return to the start. Perform all reps on one side before switching sides.

>>tip

Start off with very light weight and just do as many reps as are comfortable. Many of these exercises require strong balance and coordination. Even if you're an experienced lifter, start off as if you were a beginner and work on perfecting the movement patterns first.

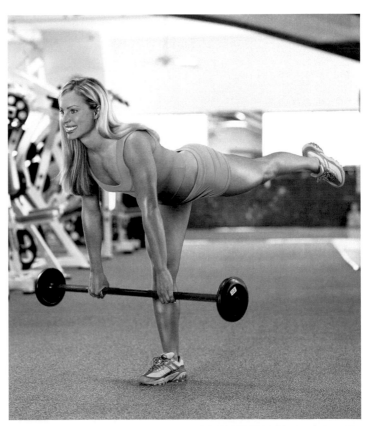

GETTING STARTED | The foundation to building a firm backside lies in a solid leg-training program. You can't train legs without enlisting the glutes, and some of the best exercises include squats, lunges and leg presses. Use these alternatives to help shape up your rear.

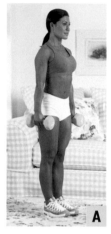
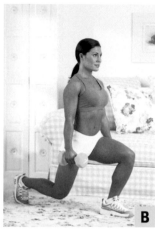
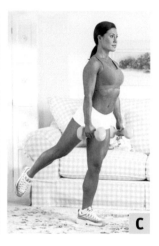

Reverse Lunge With Leg Lift

Standing erect with a dumbbell in each hand, arms by your sides (A), step back with your right leg as far as you can, bending your left knee to about 90 degrees (make sure it doesn't move past your toes). As soon as you descend into the lunge (B), contract your glutes and push through both feet to return to standing as you extend your right leg behind you without arching your low back (C). Hold for a two-count, then return to the start. Repeat for reps, alternating legs.

Single-Leg Squat to Skater's Leap

Get in a single-leg squat position with your bodyweight on your right leg, left leg raised in front of you with your knee bent. Lean forward slightly while keeping your back flat, using your arms to balance — right arm out in front of your body, left arm behind. Explosively leap sideways, squeezing your glutes and shifting all your weight onto your left leg as you land in a single-leg squat with your left arm out in front and your right arm behind. Repeat for reps back and forth, working to increase your lateral distance.

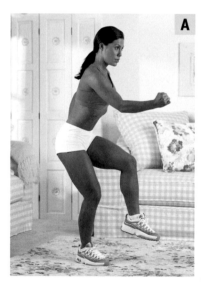
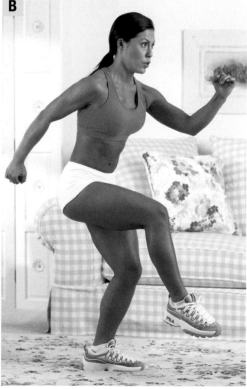

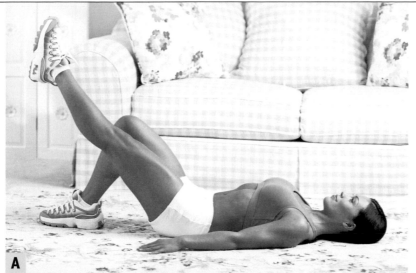

A

Single-Leg Bridge

Lie faceup on the floor with your arms down by your sides. Bend your right leg to a 90-degree angle, foot flat on the floor, keeping your left leg straight and raised 45 degrees. Press through your right heel and contract your glutes to lift your hips toward the ceiling. Hold for a count of two, then return to the start position. Repeat for reps, then switch legs.

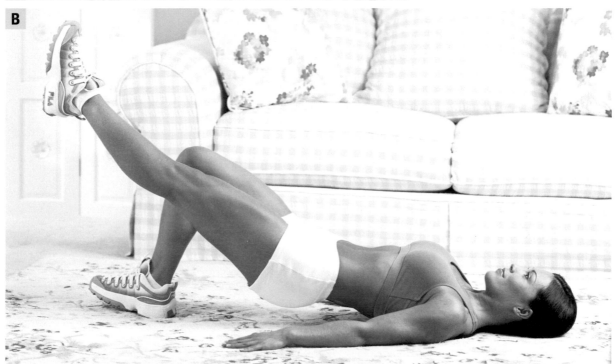

B

>>tip

The area where the hamstrings meet the glutes — called the glute-ham tie-in — needs attention, too. Squeeze through that area during leg lifts and bridging to help eradicate the flab.

At-Home Glute-Focused Routine

Exercise	Sets	Reps
Reverse Lunge With Leg Lift	3–4	12–15*
Single-Leg Squat to Skater's Leap	3–4	12–15*
Single-Leg Bridge	3–4	12–15*
*each side		

GETTING STARTED | Legs are a large muscle group that require a lot of energy when you train them. Give them their own day in your workout split, and utilize the wide range of equipment available to stay motivated and enhance your size and strength gains.

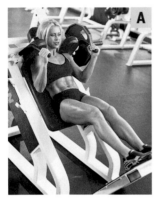
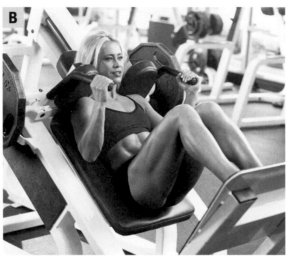

Hack Squat

Position yourself in the machine so your shoulders fit snugly under the pads, your low back and hips pressed into the backpad. With your feet shoulder-width apart near the top of the platform, unlock the safeties and straighten your legs. Bend your knees to begin the descent, moving slowly to minimize the acceleration. As your thighs come parallel to the foot platform, press through your heels as you push your hips into the pad on the way up to help stabilize your hips and low back.

Stiff-Legged Deadlift

Stand erect holding a barbell at arms' length with an overhand grip, knees slightly bent. Your hands and feet are shoulder-width apart. Looking straight ahead and keeping your bodyweight centered over your heels, hinge at the hips and push them back to lower the bar as far as is comfortable, making sure the bar doesn't drift out from your body and your back doesn't round. After holding the stretch for a moment, forcefully contract your hams and glutes to push your hips forward and raise your torso.

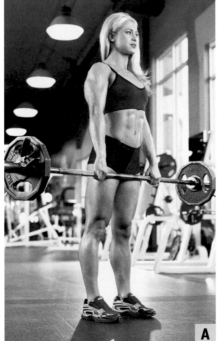
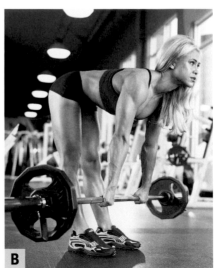

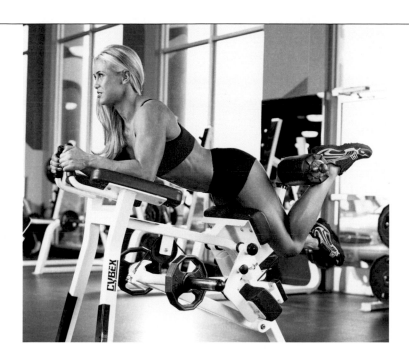

One-Leg Hamstring Curl

Position yourself in the machine so your body is at roughly a 45-degree angle, with your ankles under the rollers, your thighs resting on one set of pads and your forearms resting on another as you grasp the handles. With your back arched naturally, shoulders back and abs tight, contract your left hamstring to raise the roller in a smooth motion till it almost touches your glute. Hold for a moment and squeeze your hamstring before returning to the start position. Repeat for reps, then switch legs.

Calf Raise

Stand erect on a step, grasping a machine frame for support, and balance the balls of your feet firmly on the step's edge. (Any platform will do as long as it allows you to fully stretch your calves without your heels touching the floor.) Forcefully contract your calf muscles to raise your heels as high as you can as you rise up onto your toes. Hold the top position for a moment before slowly returning to the fully stretched position. To add resistance, grasp a dumbbell in one hand.

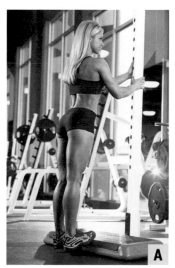 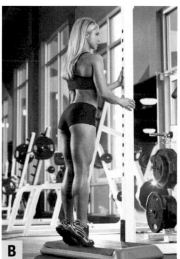

A   B

>>tip

For the sake of variety and balanced development, try going through a 12-week cycle where you start with, for example, a narrow stance on your squats and then inch your feet progressively farther apart.

Top-to-Bottom Leg Routine

Exercise	Sets	Reps
Hack Squat	4	15–20
Stiff-Legged Deadlift	4	15–20
One-Leg Hamstring Curl	4	15–20*
Calf Raise	4	15–20

*each side

upper body

Chapter SEVEN

Ultimate Upper Body

You've heard it before: There are no shortcuts to anyplace worth going. So if you want to buff up your chest, back, arms and shoulders — and enhance how your entire physique looks as a result — you must get stronger by training harder.

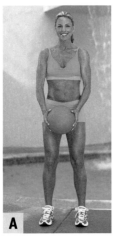

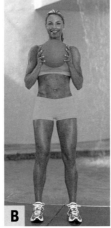

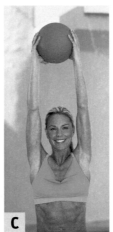

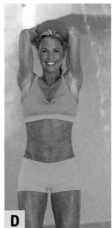

A **B** **C** **D**

Medicine-Ball Triple Threat

Stand erect with your feet about hip-width apart and the ball in your hands, arms extended down in front of you (A). Curl the ball up to your chest (B), press it overhead (C), then bend your elbows to drop it just behind your head (D). Reverse the three-step sequence and repeat for reps.

Medicine-Ball Push-Up

Get into push-up position with one hand on the ball, hands outside shoulder width. Keep the toes of both feet on the floor or hook one ankle behind the other, as shown. Execute a push-up and repeat for reps, then switch sides. To increase the difficulty, roll the ball back and forth between your hands at the top of the push-up or use two balls, one for each hand.

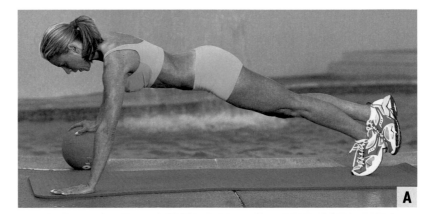

A

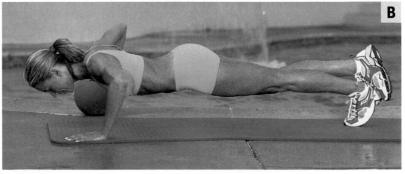

B

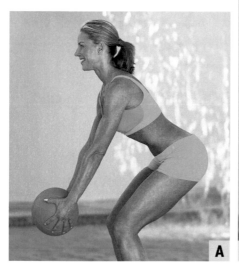

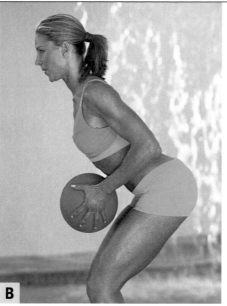

A   B

Medicine-Ball Bent-Over Row

Stand with your feet hip-width apart and your knees bent, holding the ball in both hands in front of your body with straight arms. Tighten your abs and lean forward at the hips, keeping your back flat and head neutral. Pull the ball in toward your abs while squeezing your shoulder blades together. Hold for a beat, then reverse.

Medicine-Ball Chest Toss

Lie faceup with your knees bent and feet flat on the floor, holding the ball just above your mid-chest as shown. Fully extend your arms to toss the ball into the air directly above you, catching it as it comes back down and returning it to your chest. Increase the height of the throw as you progress.

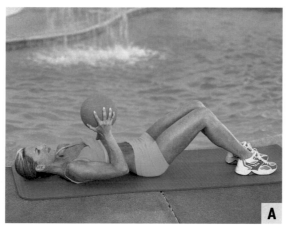

A

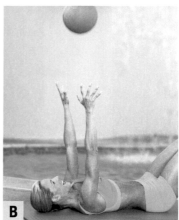

B

>>tip

Start with a 2–4-pound ball and simply work to learn the movement pattern of each exercise. As you grow more comfortable, add speed and eventually more weight.

Medicine-Ball Routine

Exercise	Sets	Reps
Medicine-Ball Triple Threat	3	10–12
Medicine-Ball Push-Up	3	10–12*
Medicine-Ball Bent-Over Row	3	10–12
Medicine-Ball Chest Toss	3	10–12

Turn this routine into a circuit by doing 15–20 reps per exercise and going through the circuit three times.
*each side

GETTING STARTED | For fast workouts and fast results, cables deliver. The continuous tension and full range of motion pump you up in a hurry. Versatile and easy to use, the cable station is a sort of "one-stop shopping" area for a resistance workout.

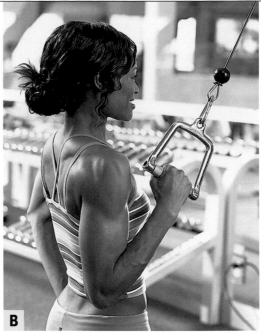

One-Arm Pulldown

Set the pulley to the topmost setting and clip on a D-handle. Grasp the handle with your right hand so your palm faces forward, arm extended. Kneel down, torso erect, with your right shoulder just to the left of the pulley. Keep your body stationary as you pull the handle down and to the outside of your shoulder, bringing your elbow toward your side as you turn your palm in and squeeze your shoulder blade toward your spine. Slowly straighten your arm and return to the start. Repeat for reps, then switch arms.

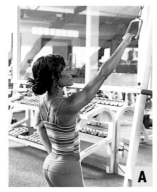

A B

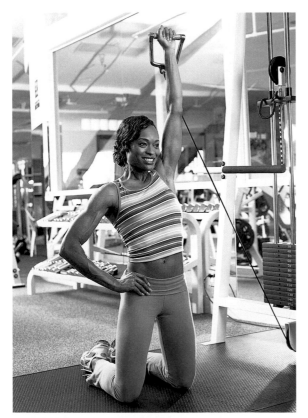

One-Arm Cable Overhead Press

Set a cable pulley at the bottom position and clip on a D-handle. Grasp the handle in your left hand, palm facing forward, and kneel sideways to and about 6–8 inches from the weight stack and several inches in front of it, torso erect. Raise your left arm so your elbow is bent 90 degrees, with your upper arm parallel to the floor. Press the handle overhead until your arm is fully extended, but don't lock out your elbow. Slowly lower to the start. Repeat for reps, then switch arms.

Cable-Ready Routine

Exercise	Sets	Reps
One-Arm Pulldown	3	8–12*
One-Arm Cable Overhead Press	3	8–12*
Rope Pressdown	3	8–12
Seated Cable Concentration Curl	3	8–12*
Cable Crossover	3	8–12
*each side		

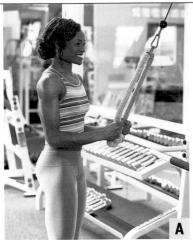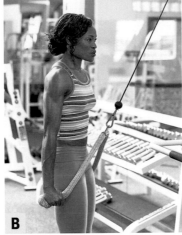

Rope Pressdown

Set a cable pulley to the topmost position and clip on the rope attachment. Face the pulley and grasp one end of the rope in each hand. Step back a few inches to create some tension in the cable and bend your elbows so your forearms are parallel to the floor. Keeping your upper arms still, squeeze your tri's to straighten your arms until your hands are alongside your thighs. Follow the same path to return to the start.

Seated Cable Concentration Curl

Set a cable pulley to the bottom setting and clip on a D-handle. Place a bench perpendicular to and a few feet away from the weight stack. Sit down and grasp the handle in your right hand. Lean forward with your back flat and straighten your right arm, placing the back of your upper arm against the inside of your right thigh close to your knee with your palm facing upward. Curl the handle toward your shoulder, squeezing your biceps hard at the top. Repeat for reps, then switch arms.

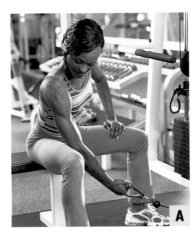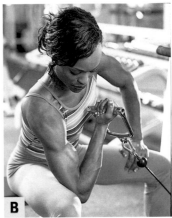

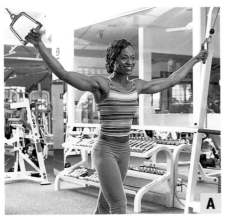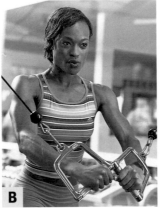

Cable Crossover

Move both pulleys to the top position and attach D-handles. Stand in the center of the cable tower and grasp a handle in each hand with your palms facing forward, arms extended out to your sides. Take a step forward with your right foot and lean slightly forward from the hips, back flat. Keeping a slight bend in your elbows, sweep your arms down and in front of you until your hands meet in front of your lower chest. Reverse the motion until your elbows come just above shoulder height.

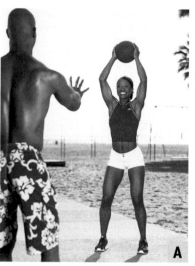
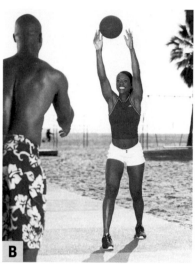

Medicine-Ball Overhead Throw

Standing erect with your feet shoulder-width apart and knees slightly bent, hold the medicine ball above your head with your arms fully extended. Reach backward, moving the ball behind your head. Without overly arching your back, throw the ball to a partner or against a wall, releasing the ball when it's just above your head.

Medicine-Ball Standing Chest Push-Pass

With your feet shoulder-width apart and knees slightly bent, stand erect opposite a partner or a wall. Hold the medicine ball to your chest, elbows pointing straight out to your sides, and throw it to your partner in a push-pass action. The pass should be explosive as if you're passing a basketball. Don't overextend your elbows.

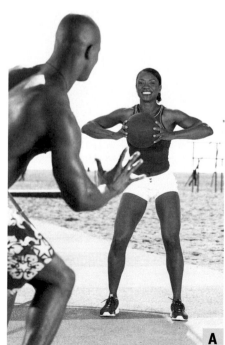
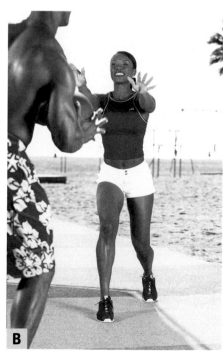

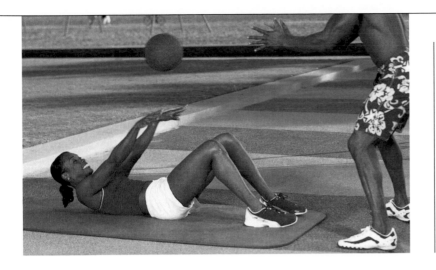

Medicine-Ball Pullover Throw

Lie faceup with your knees bent and feet flat on the floor, holding a medicine ball directly over your chest with your arms almost fully extended. Have your partner stand about 5–10 feet away. Lower the ball behind your head as far as you can, touching the floor if possible. From this position, crunch up and throw the ball toward your partner, releasing it when your arms are over your chest and midsection. Pause at the top so you can catch the ball before returning to the floor.

Medicine-Ball Lateral Throw

With your partner standing about 20 feet to your right side, stand erect with your feet shoulder-width apart, knees slightly bent and your left foot just ahead of your right. Hold the medicine ball with both hands directly in front of you. Keep your arms extended and parallel to the floor. Swing the ball as far to the left as you can, allowing your hips to turn with your arms. Immediately swing the ball to your right and throw it to your partner. Complete your reps for one side, then switch sides.

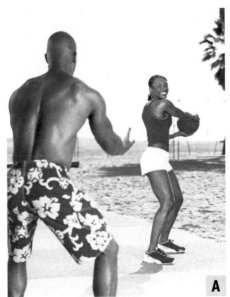

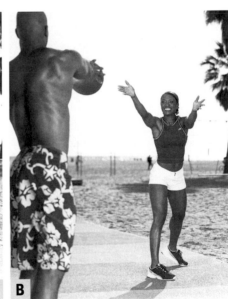

A   **B**

>>tip

Warm up before the workout, stretch afterward and be careful not to do too much too soon. Beginners shouldn't exceed 80 reps per session. Do just one plyo routine each week.

Medicine-Ball Partnered Routine

Exercise	Sets	Reps	Rest
Medicine-Ball Overhead Throw	2–3	8	2 min.
Medicine-Ball Standing Chest Push-Pass	2–3	8	2 min.
Medicine-Ball Pullover Throw	2–3	8	2 min.
Medicine-Ball Lateral Throw	1–2	8	1.5 min.*

Start with the lightest medicine ball available (2–4 pounds) and slowly progress to heavier ones. In the beginning, perform only 1–2 sets per exercise and slowly work up to 2–3.
*each side

GETTING STARTED | When time is tight, superset pairs of exercises to speed things up and increase intensity. Once you finish the first movement, immediately begin the second. Each time you train, reverse the order within each pair of exercises. Warm up first.

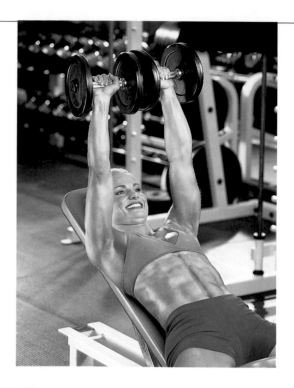

Incline Dumbbell Press

Performing a press on the incline bench requires that you align yourself and the weights properly. Lie faceup on a bench set to a 30–45-degree incline, feet on the floor, your chest arched upward and abs tight to stabilize your body. Using a similar tempo and range of motion as on a flat-bench press, press the weights directly over your upper chest and squeeze at the top, then return under full control so your upper arms dip just past parallel to the floor. Don't go any deeper or you risk injury to your shoulder joints.

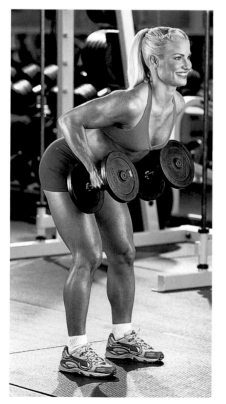

Bent-Over Dumbbell Row

Lean forward with your feet about shoulder-width apart, knees slightly bent, a slight arch in your lower back. Start with the weights down in front of your legs, then squeeze your shoulder blades together and pull the weights up to your sides, keeping your elbows close to your body. Control the return.

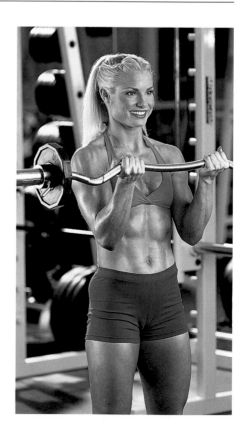

EZ-Bar Curl

Take a shoulder-width, underhand grip on the EZ-bar and stand erect, abs tight and knees soft. Curl the bar toward your shoulders, squeeze and lower under control, stopping just short of full extension. Keep your elbows by your sides throughout and avoid swinging your body.

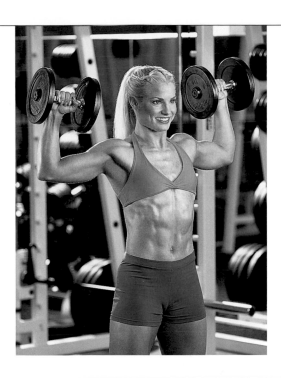

Standing Overhead Dumbbell Press

With a dumbbell in each hand, stand erect in front of a mirror, knees soft and abs tight. Lift the weights so your upper arms are about parallel to the floor, elbows bent 90 degrees. Press the weights overhead, bringing them together at the top. Don't lock out your elbows. Reverse in a controlled manner.

>>tip

By doing primarily compound (multi-joint) exercises, you work more than one muscle group at a time, which brings your muscles to fatigue faster and reduces time spent in the gym.

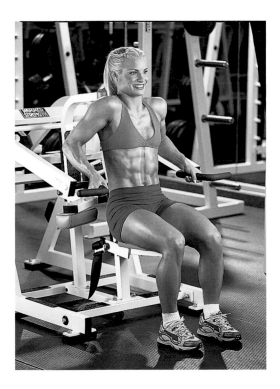

Machine Dip

Sit in the machine with your back and hips flush against the pads, feet flat on the floor. Grasp the handles at waist level, palms facing in and elbows pointing backward, and squeeze through your triceps to push them down to full arm extension. Control the return, keeping your shoulders down and back flat.

Superset Upper-Body Routine

Exercise	Sets	Reps
Incline Dumbbell Press —superset with—	3	8–12
Bent-Over Dumbbell Row	3	8–12
Standing Overhead Dumbbell Press —superset with—	2	8–12
Bent-Over Lateral Raise	2	8–12
EZ-Bar Curl —superset with—	2	8–12
Machine Dip	2	8–12

Do each of the paired exercises back-to-back with no rest in between.

GETTING STARTED | In most cases, a muscle's action can be classified as a push or pull movement. Grouping workouts in this manner minimizes the risk of injury and imbalance around your joints. Do each workout once a week, leaving at least a day between sessions.

Pec-Deck Flye

Sit upright and fully supported at the machine, feet flat on the floor, grasping the handles with your palms facing in. Your wrists, elbows and shoulders should all be in line. Squeeze your chest to bring the handles together in front of you, keeping your elbows up and slightly bent. Lightly touch the handles together, then slowly return to the start.

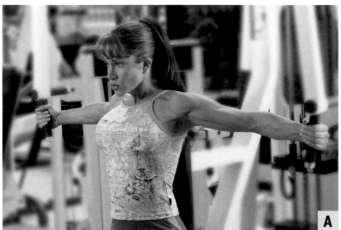
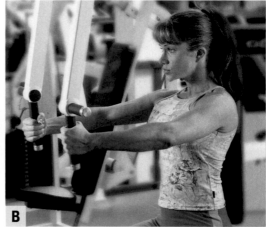

Lying EZ-Bar Extension

Lie faceup on a flat bench and hold an EZ-bar or barbell over your upper chest with your arms straight. Bending only your elbows, slowly lower the bar toward your forehead, stopping before it touches your head. Contract your triceps to push the bar back up to the start.

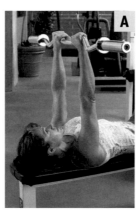
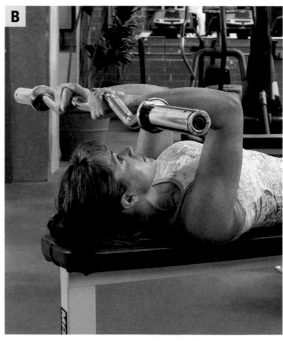

Upper-Body Push Routine

Exercise	Sets	Reps
Dumbbell Bench Press	3	12–15
Pec-Deck Flye	3	12–15
Standing Overhead Dumbbell Press	3	12–15
Front Dumbbell Raise	3	12–15
Lying EZ-Bar Extension	3	12–15

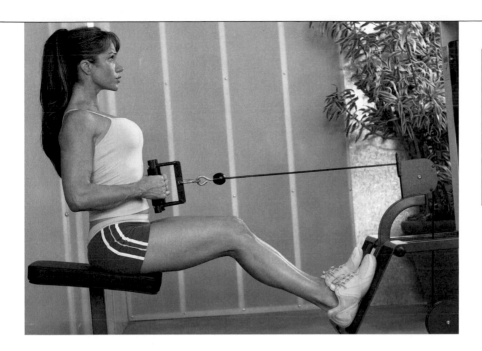

Seated Cable Row

Sit erect at a cable row machine with your knees slightly bent and your shoulders down and back, arms extended in front of you. Keeping your elbows close to your sides, pull the handle toward your abs, squeezing your shoulder blades together. Pause, then resist the pull of the cable on the return.

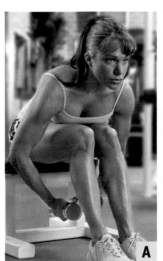
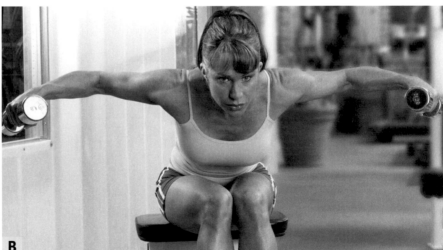

Bent-Over Lateral Raise

Sit at the end of a flat bench holding a dumbbell in each hand; lean forward so your chest rests on your thighs and the weights hang under your legs. Keeping your back flat and elbows slightly bent, slowly raise the dumbbells up and out to your sides, keeping them in your peripheral vision to make sure you're in the correct plane of motion. Lead with your elbows, not your hands.

Upper-Body Pull Routine

Exercise	Sets	Reps
Pull-Up	3	12–15
Seated Cable Row	3	12–15
Bent-Over Lateral Raise	3	12–15
Concentration Curl	3	12–15*

*each side

lower body

Chapter EIGHT

Landmark Lower Body

If you have your share of typical trouble spots, you probably dream of tight, toned thighs and shapely glutes. Wake up and use these workouts in conjunction with the upper-body routines in Chapter 7 to create a truly awe-inspiring physique.

Depth Jump

Do this advanced exercise early in your workout. Start from a "ready" position atop a box, sturdy chair or other stable surface about 12–15 inches high (A). Step off the platform (do not jump off) and, as soon as you hit the floor (B), explosively jump up as high as possible (C). Step back onto the platform and repeat for reps. Minimize the time you spend on the floor to improve your rate of force development.

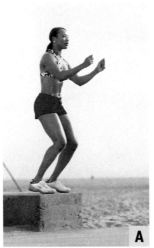

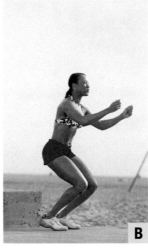

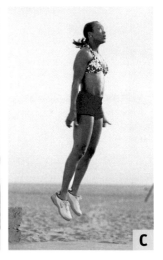

180-Degree Jump

Standing erect, take off using a two-foot jump (A), then rotate in midair 180 degrees (B). Land on both feet, arms outstretched, and hold for two seconds (C). Repeat in the opposite direction to complete one rep.

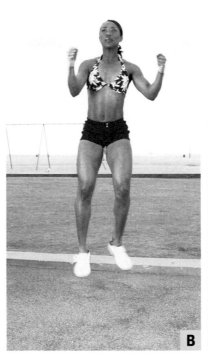

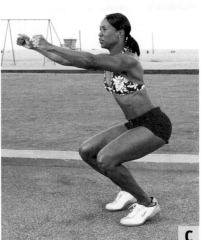

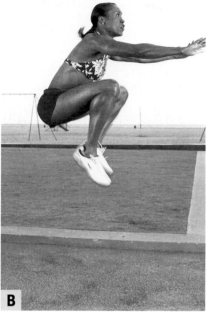

Tuck Jump

Start from a "ready" position, arms outstretched, and jump up as high as you can, bringing both knees as high as possible to your chest. As you land, go right into the next jump, minimizing the amount of time your feet touch the floor.

A   **B**

Bounding

Think of this exercise as an aggressive type of skipping. You simply skip, bringing your body as high and as far forward as possible, leading with your forward knee. Try to minimize floor contact time.

A   **B**

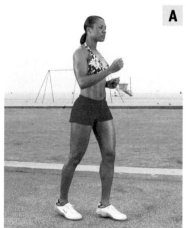

Plyometric Lower-Body Routine

Exercise	Sets	Reps
Bounding	1–3	20 yds. total
Depth Jump	2–3	6
Tuck Jump	4–6	3
180-Degree Jump	2–3	6

Start by doing the least amount of sets suggested and slowly increase as you progress. Rest 2–3 minutes between sets.

GETTING STARTED | Use this routine to blast your lower half in less than 30 minutes using supersets. The intensity is high, so you may need at least 48 hours of recovery time before training legs again. Check the index to review any exercises you're unfamiliar with.

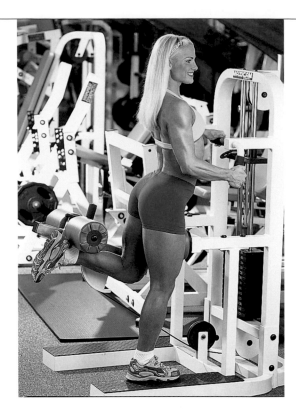

One-Leg Hamstring Curl

Adjust the ankle rollers so they hit just above your Achilles. Stand erect and curl one leg at a time to just past 90 degrees, squeezing your hamstring and glute at the top. Return to the start but stop the motion before the weight touches the stack. Repeat for reps, then switch legs.

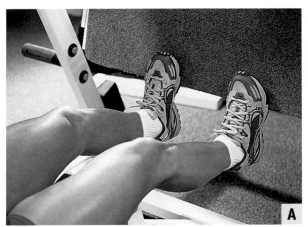
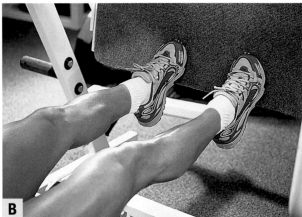

Leg-Press Calf Raise

With the same setup you use for the leg press, place the balls of your feet at the lower edge of the platform at about hip width. Fully extend your legs to unhook the safeties. Keeping your knees slightly bent, press the weight up by extending your ankles and contracting your calves. Lower as far as possible, getting a good stretch.

Weighted Step-Up

Standing erect with dumbbells at your sides, plant one foot on top of a step. Push through the heel of that foot to lift your body, squeezing through your glutes, until you're standing erect atop the step. Reverse the movement to return to the start position, touching your back foot to the floor only briefly. Repeat for reps, then switch legs.

>>tip

Warm up for five minutes to help improve your focus and reduce your risk of injury. Do the workout in the order presented — from large muscles to smaller ones.

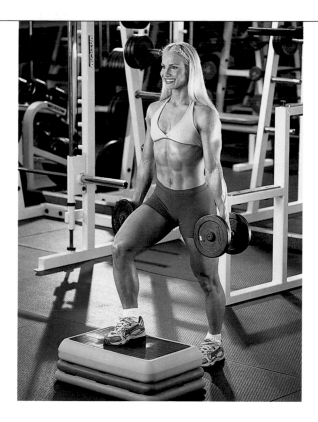

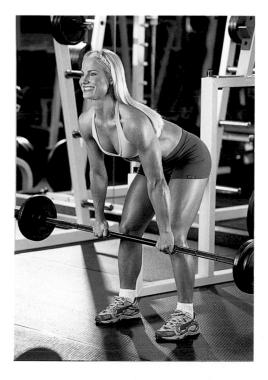

Romanian Deadlift

Using an overhand or staggered grip, stand erect with your chest high, back slightly arched and knees slightly bent, feet hip-width apart. As you lean forward from your hips, slide the bar down your legs. Reverse the motion as you push your hips forward and squeeze your glutes.

30-Minute
Lower-Body Routine

Exercise	Sets	Reps
Back Squat	3	10–15
—superset with—		
Romanian Deadlift	3	10–15
Weighted Step-Up	2	10–15*
—superset with—		
One-Leg Hamstring Curl	2	10–15*
Leg Press	2	10–15
—superset with—		
Leg-Press Calf Raise	2	10–15
Seated Calf Raise	2	10–15
—superset with—		
Crunch	2	10–15

*each side
Rest one minute between supersets.

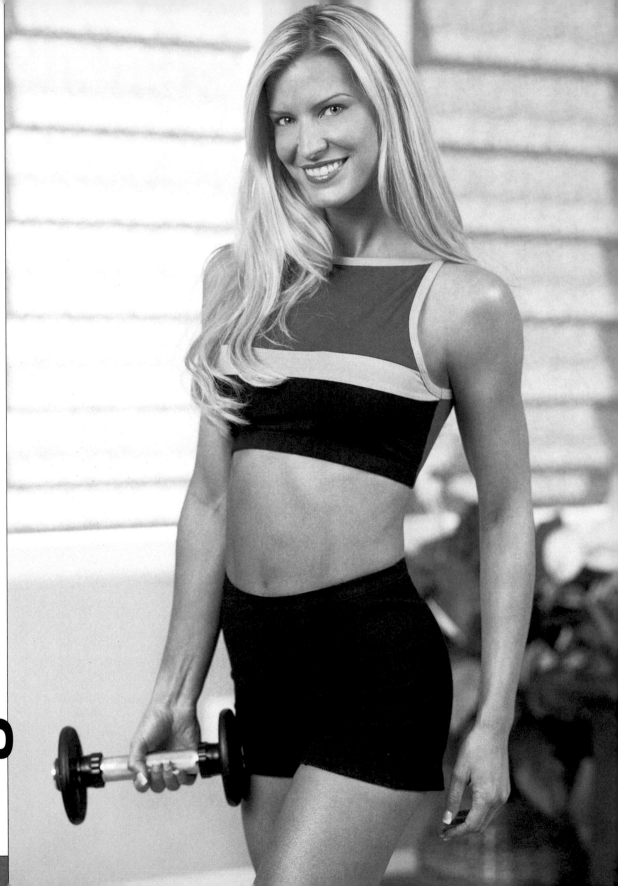

beginners

Chapter NINE

Getting Started

Even the best-built bodies started at the beginning and hit plateaus along the way. These workout programs can introduce you to weight training, serve as a segue between ability levels or shock your muscles when your progress has stalled.

WORKOUT 78

GETTING STARTED | If you prefer training at home, resistance bands are an inexpensive alternative to investing in a full spectrum of weights or jumping into a gym membership. Do this workout twice a week, building up to doing more sets and/or using greater resistance.

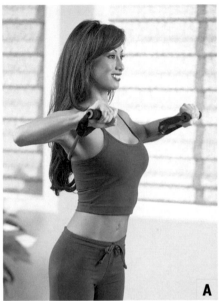
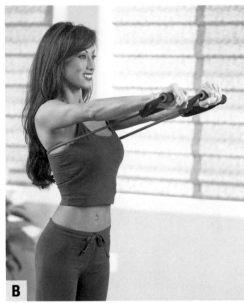

A **B**

Resistance-Band Chest Press

Stand erect, feet hip-width apart and knees slightly bent, with the band behind your upper-middle back. Shorten the band so you feel some resistance in the start position, elbows bent 90 degrees. Press straight out in front of you at shoulder level, then return to the start.

Resistance-Band Back Row

Sit on the floor with your legs outstretched, knees bent slightly and back erect. Loop the band around your feet to provide some resistance in the start position, arms out in front of you. Pull the handles toward your ribs, bringing your elbows behind the plane of your back and squeezing your shoulder blades together.

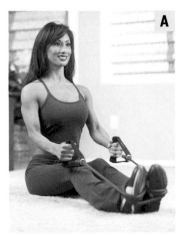
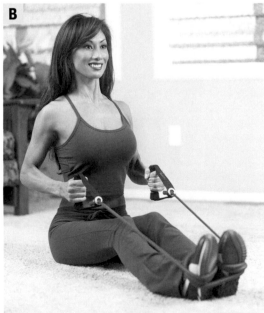

A **B**

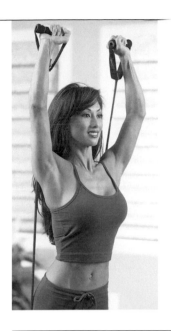

Resistance-Band Overhead Press

Stand erect, feet hip-width apart, with the band under your feet and positioned behind your body. Press up from your shoulders to full arm extension without locking out your elbows.

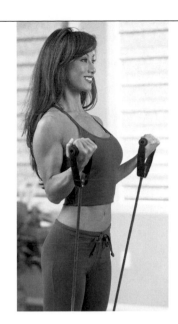

Resistance-Band Biceps Curl

Stand erect, feet hip-width apart, with the band under your feet and hands down by your sides. Curl up toward your shoulders, keeping your elbows tight to your sides.

Resistance-Band Squat

Stand erect, feet hip-width apart, with the band under your feet; grasp the handles outside your shoulders with the band behind your arms. Descend into a squat, keeping your back flat. Press through your heels to stand back up.

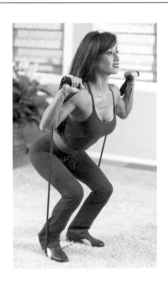

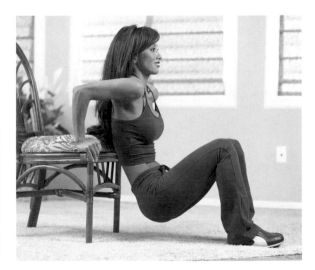

Dips Using a Chair

Sit at the edge of a chair, grasping the edges next to your hips, feet flat on the floor. Move your glutes just off the chair and descend to a 90-degree bend in your elbows, then press back up.

At-Home Beginner Routine

Exercise	Sets	Reps
Resistance-Band Chest Press	1–2	12–15
Resistance-Band Back Row	1–2	12–15
Resistance-Band Overhead Press	1–2	12–15
Resistance-Band Biceps Curl	1–2	12–15
Dips using a Chair	1–2	12–15
Resistance-Band Squat	1–2	12–15
Crunch	1–2	12–15
Calf Raise	1–2	12–15

>>tip

Even though you're working with bands, make sure the resistance is moderate to hard intensity. This shouldn't feel easy.

GETTING STARTED | This 12-week beginner's program is divided into three stages of four weeks each. Each portion of the program introduces you to new exercises and training techniques as well as heavier workloads, including cardio exercise, in a safe and effective manner.

STAGE 1: Week 1

Do one set of 10–12 reps of the exercises listed below with either your bodyweight or very light weight. Don't push to the point of struggling to complete your reps; beginning slowly gives you time to concentrate on form and ensures you don't get so sore that you give up. Weight-train three times this week, allowing a day of recovery between sessions. Do two 20-minute cardio workouts, training at a comfortable level.

Exercises	
Plié Squat	Leg-Press Calf Raise
Stiff-Legged Deadlift	Exercise-Ball Push-Up
Leg Press	Incline Dumbbell Press

Week 2

Add one set to each exercise and increase reps to 12–15. Cardio stays the same.

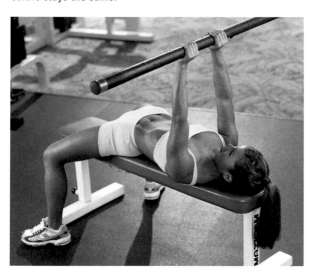

Close-Grip Bench Press

Lie faceup on a flat bench, grasp a Body Bar or barbell inside shoulder width and hold it just above the center of your chest, elbows pointing out to your sides. Contract your chest to press the bar directly upward until your arms are fully extended, elbows unlocked. Slowly lower the bar back to the start position.

Week 3

Stay with two sets and increase reps to 15–20. Extend one of your cardio sessions to 25 minutes.

Week 4

Stay with two sets, drop the reps back down to 12–15 and increase the weights to the point where you reach momentary muscle failure somewhere in this range. Cardio stays the same.

STAGE 2: Week 5

This week you'll start following a split routine instead of training your entire body each day you work out, and you'll learn some new exercises as well. You can train on consecutive days as long as you don't train a sore bodypart. Add in another day of cardio, doing 20 minutes twice a week and 30 minutes the third day. During your short sessions, increase intensity so the workouts feel challenging. For the 30-minute session, keep it comfortable. You can do cardio either on your off days or on the same days you weight-train. In the latter case, do your weight-training first, when you're fresh and strong.

Day 1: Chest, Triceps, Deltoids	
Do three sets of 10–12 reps.	
Incline Dumbbell Press	
Exercise-Ball Push-Up (with lower legs on ball)	
Close-Grip Bench Press	
Straight-Bar Pressdown	
Dumbbell Upright Row	
Lateral Raise	
Day 2: Legs	
Do three sets of 12–15 reps.	
Back Squat	Lying Leg Curl
Stiff-Legged Deadlift	Calf Raise
Front Lunge	
Day 3: Back, Biceps, Abs	
Do three sets of 10–12 reps.	
Lat Pulldown	Reverse Crunch
One-Arm Dumbbell Row	Cross-Body Crunch
EZ-Bar Preacher Curl	
Hammer Curl	

Weeks 6–7

Keep the same cardio, weight, sets and reps from Week 5.

Week 8

Add weight and drop the reps to 8–10. Do push-ups on your toes instead of on the exercise ball. For cardio, add another five minutes to your short sessions, so you'll now be doing two 25-minute sessions and one 30-minute session per week.

STAGE 3: Week 9

Although you'll keep your bodypart splits the same, you'll swap their order and once again incorporate some new exercises into your training, which will increase the total amount of work you do. Do two sets of 12–15 reps for each exercise. Cardio stays the same.

Day 1: Back, Biceps, Abs
Assisted Pull-Up
Seated Cable Row (wide overhand grip)
One-Arm Dumbbell Row
EZ-Bar Curl
Supinating Dumbbell Curl
Machine Preacher Curl
Hands-Overhead Crunch
Reverse Crunch

Day 2: Chest, Triceps, Deltoids
Push-Up
Incline Dumbbell Press
Barbell Bench Press
Pec-Deck Flye
Lying Dumbbell Extension
Dumbbell Kickback
Seated Military Press
Y, T & I

Day 3: Legs
Front Squat
Back Lunge
Leg Press
Weighted Step-Up
Lying Leg Curl
Stiff-Legged Deadlift
Leg-Press Calf Raise
Decline-Bench Crunch

Week 10

Your bodypart split, weights and reps stay the same from Week 9. Change the following: Of all the exercises you now know, choose four for legs, one for calves and three for all other bodyparts. Do three sets of each. For cardio, do two 25-minute sessions and two 35-minute sessions.

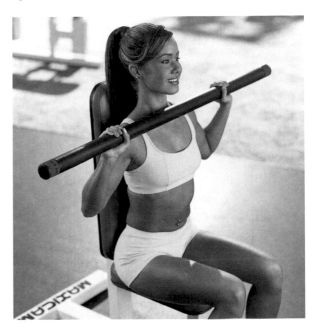

Seated Military Press

Sit erect holding a Body Bar or barbell in front of your neck just outside shoulder width, elbows pointing out to your sides. Press the bar overhead to just short of elbow lockout.

Week 11

Everything stays the same this week, except you'll change the order in which you do your exercises. If you usually start with cable rows for back, instead begin with pull-ups or an exercise you haven't done in a while. Cardio stays the same.

Week 12

Everything stays the same, though you continue to change the order of your exercises. Cardio stays the same.

GETTING STARTED | Along with having some fun, patience, practice and the correct information will transform your beginning weeks of weight training into a positive and successful experience. Train three times a week; in weeks 7–12, alternate upper- and lower-body routines.

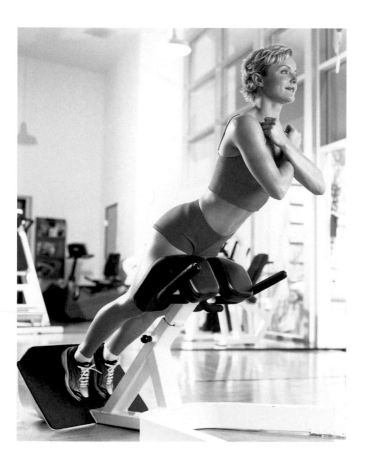

Back Extension

With your feet together at the top edge of the footplate and your thighs on the pads, start with your body in a straight line, arms crossed over your chest. Without rounding your back, hinge at the hips to lower your torso toward the floor. Squeeze through your low back and glutes to return to the start.

Seated Calf Raise
(not shown)

Sit in the machine with your back straight, abs tight and balls of your feet at the edge of the foot platform. The thigh pad should rest snugly just above your knees. Using a smooth motion, rise up onto your toes as high as possible and pause, then lower your heels as far as you can for a good stretch. Point your toes in or out for variation.

Weeks 1–6: Total Body

Exercise	Sets	Reps
Plié Squat	2	10–15
Stationary Dumbbell Lunge	2	10–15*
Machine Row	2	10–15
Push-Up	2	10–15
Incline Dumbbell Press	2	10–15
Lateral Raise	2	10–15
Standing Dumbbell Curl	2	10–15
Straight-Bar Pressdown	2	10–15
Calf Raise	2	10–15
Crunch (or Reverse Crunch)^	2	10–15
Back Extension	2	10–15

*each side ^Alternate with the reverse crunch every other workout.

Weeks 7–12: Upper Body

Exercise	Sets	Reps
One-Arm Dumbbell Row	2	10–15*
Machine Row	2	10–15
Push-Up	2	10–15
Incline Dumbbell Press	2	10–15
Dumbbell Upright Row	2	10–15
Incline Dumbbell Curl	2	10–15
Rope Pressdown	2	10–15
Crunch	2	10–15
Back Extension	2	10–15

*each side

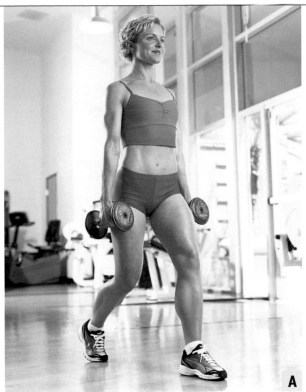

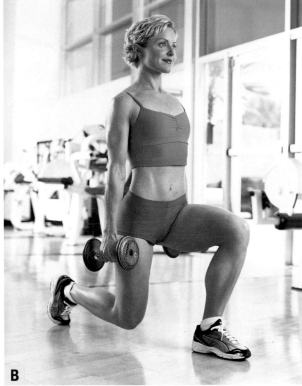

A **B**

Stationary Dumbbell Lunge

Standing erect holding dumbbells alongside your thighs, take a step forward and firmly plant your foot in the start position. Keeping your chest lifted and feet facing forward, lower your body until your back knee nearly touches the floor, being careful not to let your front knee extend past your toes. Press back up through both thighs, and repeat for reps before switching legs. Stay in place with both feet on the floor.

Adductor/Abductor Machine
(not shown)

Sit in the machine with your back and thighs flush against the seat, knees bent and feet on the footplates. In the adductor machine, you start with your legs apart and squeeze them together to work your inner thighs; in the abductor machine, you start with your legs together and push them apart to train your outer thighs. Keep the motion smooth and controlled.

>>**tip**

Use a smooth, controlled movement to lift a weight through a full range of motion. Choose a level of resistance that makes the last few reps of an exercise very challenging.

Weeks 7–12: Lower Body

Exercise	Sets	Reps
Plié Squat	2	10–15
Stationary Dumbbell Lunge	2	10–15*
Leg Extension	2	10–15
Lying Leg Curl	2	10–15
Adductor Machine^ —superset with—	2	10–15
Abductor Machine^	2	10–15
Seated Calf Raise	2	10–15

*each side
^Do these exercises back-to-back with no rest in between. Repeat for sets.

full body

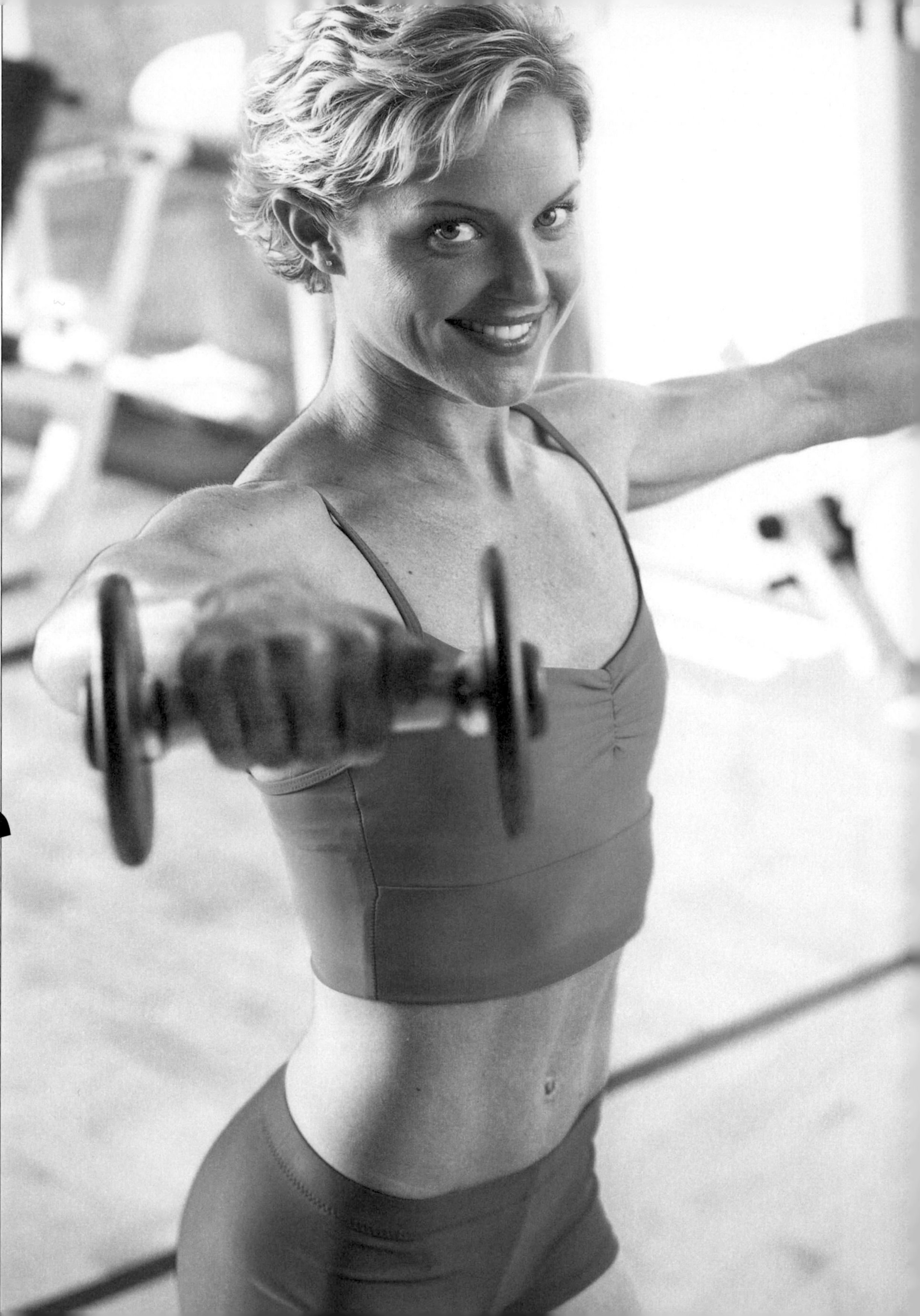

Chapter TEN

Putting It Together

Building a fit, athletic physique isn't a simple task. We make the process a bit easier, giving you everything you need in cheat-sheet form so you can accomplish your goals without having to manipulate all the variables yourself.

GETTING STARTED | This eight-week program emphasizes muscle-shaping and -building plus fat loss. Each time out, change the exercises, how long you rest between sets or how much weight you lift. Add 2.5–5 pounds if you can do another two reps two workouts in a row.

Fire-It-Up Training Split

Day	Workout
Monday	Lower Body, Cardio
Tuesday	Upper Body, Core
Wednesday	Rest
Thursday	Lower Body, Core
Friday	Upper Body, Cardio
Saturday	Cardio
Sunday	Rest

Cardio Interval Training

Do 25–35 minutes of cardio training 3–6 times a week. The activity you choose doesn't matter, as long as you follow an interval program that keeps your heart rate up and varies your intensity levels.

30-Minute Workout	
3 minutes	Warm-up
24 minutes	Intervals: Work at 85%–90% of your target heart rate for one minute, then recover at 65%–70% for two minutes. Repeat.
3 minutes	Cool-down

Barbell Bench Press

Lie faceup on a flat bench, grasp a barbell a little wider than shoulder width and hold it slightly above the center of your chest, elbows pointing out to your sides. Contract your chest to press the bar directly upward until your arms are fully extended, elbows unlocked. Slowly lower the bar back to the start position.

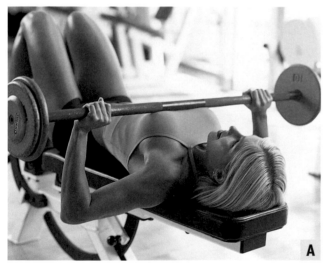

A

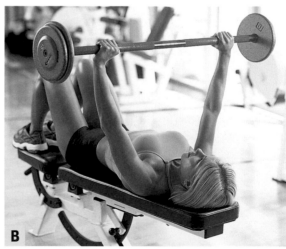

B

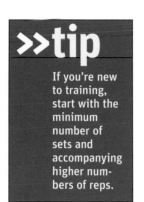
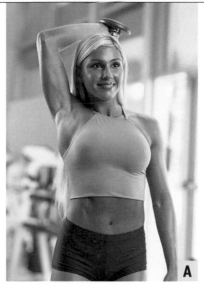

A

One-Arm Overhead Dumbbell Extension

Stand erect with your shoulders rolled back and down. Grasp a dumbbell so your pinky touches the plate on that side, and position your hand behind your head. Extend your arm overhead, squeeze at the top, then bend your elbow to bring the weight down behind your head under control. Make sure your elbow points upward and your upper arm stays over your ear throughout the exercise. Repeat for reps, then switch sides.

B

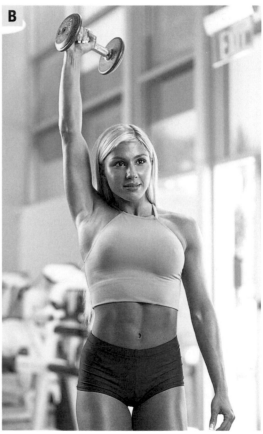

Upper-Body Routine

Exercise	Sets	Reps
Bent-Over Barbell Row	2–3	12, 10, 8
Barbell Bench Press	2–3	12, 10, 8
Lat Pulldown	2–3	12, 10, 8
Incline Dumbbell Press	2–3	12, 10, 8
Standing Overhead Dumbbell Press	2–3	12, 10, 8
Lateral Raise	2–3	12, 10, 8
Supinating Dumbbell Curl	2–3	12, 10, 8
One-Arm Overhead Dumbbell Extension	2–3	12, 10, 8*

*each side

Lower-Body Routine

Exercise	Sets	Reps
Back Squat	3–4	12, 12, 10, 8
Romanian Deadlift	3–4	12, 12, 10, 8
Walking Lunge	3–4	12, 12, 10, 8*
Weighted Step-Up	3–4	12, 12, 10, 8*
Leg Press	3–4	12, 12, 10, 8
Seated Calf Raise	3–4	12, 12, 10, 8

*each side

Core Routine

Exercise	WEEKS 1–2 Sets	WEEKS 1–2 Reps	WEEKS 3–6 Sets	WEEKS 3–6 Reps	WEEKS 7–8 Sets	WEEKS 7–8 Reps
Crunch	1	15–30	2	15–30	3	15–30
Cross-Body Crunch	1	15–30*	2	15–30*	3	15–30*
Exercise-Ball Crunch	1	15–30	2	15–30	3	15–30
Reverse Crunch	1	15–30	2	15–30	3	15–30
Exercise-Ball Opposite Arm/Leg Lift	1	15–30*	2	15–30*	3	15–30*
Seated Exercise-Ball Bridge	1	15–30	2	15–30	3	15–30

*each side

GETTING STARTED | In this 12-week program you'll gradually increase your weights and decrease the reps to build strength. For efficiency, most exercises are grouped in super-sets or tri-sets, in which you do two or three different exercises back to back without rest.

Day 1: Lower-Body Routine

Exercise	WEEKS 1–5 Sets	Reps	WEEKS 6–10 Sets	Reps	WEEKS 11–12 Sets	Reps
Back Squat —superset with—	3	12	3	9	3	6
Incline Dumbbell Press	3	12	3	9	3	6
Front Lunge —superset with—	3	12*	3	9*	3	6*
Lat Pulldown	3	12	3	9	3	6
Weighted Step-Up —superset with—	3	12*	3	9*	3	6*
Bench Dip	3	12	3	9	3	6
Romanian Deadlift —superset with—	3	12	3	9	3	6
Dumbbell Upright Row	3	12	3	9	3	6
Calf Raise —superset with—	3	12	3	9	3	6
Seated Alternating Dumbbell Curl	3	12	3	9	3	6

*each side

Day 2: Chest & Shoulders Routine

Exercise	WEEKS 1–5 Sets	Reps	WEEKS 6–10 Sets	Reps	WEEKS 11–12 Sets	Reps
Barbell Bench Press —superset with—	3	12	3	9	3	6
Good Morning	3	12	3	9	3	6
Leg Press —superset with—	3	12	3	9	3	6
Alternating Front and Lateral Raise^	3	12	3	9	3	6
Incline Dumbbell Flye —tri-set with—	3	12	3	9	3	6
Incline Dumbbell Curl	3	12	3	9	3	6
Seated Overhead Dumbbell Press	3	12	3	9	3	6
Cable Crossover —superset with—	3	12	3	9	3	6
Seated Cable Row	3	12	3	9	3	6
Crunch —superset with—	3	12	3	9	3	6
Cross-Body Crunch	3	12*	3	9*	3	6*

*each side ^See exercise description on page 62, but use dumbbells.

Day 3: Back & Arms Routine

Exercise	WEEKS 1–5 Sets	Reps	WEEKS 6–10 Sets	Reps	WEEKS 11–12 Sets	Reps
Assisted Wide-Grip Pull-Up —tri-set with—	3	12	3	9	3	6
Assisted Close-Grip Pull-Up^	3	12	3	9	3	6
Weighted Step-Up	3	12*	3	9*	3	6*
Close-Grip Bench Press —superset with—	3	12	3	9	3	6
Supinating Dumbbell Curl	3	12	3	9	3	6
Leg Extension —superset with—	3	12	3	9	3	6
Lying Leg Curl	3	12	3	9	3	6
One-Arm Dumbbell Row —superset with—	3	12*	3	9*	3	6*
Dumbbell Kickback	3	12*	3	9*	3	6*
EZ-Bar Curl —superset with—	3	12	3	9	3	6
Lying EZ-Bar Extension	3	12	3	9	3	6
Back Extension —superset with—	3	12	3	9	3	6
Reverse Decline Crunch	3	12	3	9	3	6

*each side ^Perform just like the wide-grip pull-up, but bring your hands closer together.

Day 4: Core Routine

Exercise	WEEKS 1–5 Sets	Reps	WEEKS 6–10 Sets	Reps	WEEKS 11–12 Sets	Reps
Exercise-Ball Crunch —superset with—	3	12	3	9	3	6
Exercise-Ball Back Extension	3	12	3	9	3	6
Wide-Grip Standing Lat Pulldown —superset with—	3	12	3	9	3	6
Close-Grip Standing Lat Pulldown	3	12	3	9	3	6
Walking Lunge	3	12*	3	9*	3	6*
Rope Pressdown	3	12	3	9	3	6
Hammer Curl	3	12	3	9	3	6

*each side

>>tip

Train every other day, doing the workouts in order. Select a weight that makes the last few reps of each exercise very challenging, though you should still be able to complete them with good form.

Standing Lat Pulldown

Stand erect at the lat pull-down machine with your feet about hip-width apart and knees slightly bent. Grasp the bar so your hands are just wider than shoulder width. Begin with straightened and elevated arms, then hinge at the shoulders to press the bar straight down to your thighs. Return under control, allowing the bar to move above the level of your head.

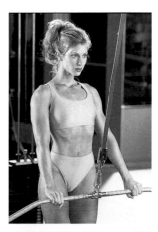

92-93

EZ-Bar Curl

Take a hip-width stance, knees slightly bent, bar down in front of your thighs. Curl the weight up while keeping your upper arms in place alongside your torso. At the top, concentrate on getting a good squeeze before lowering the bar under control. Don't lock out your elbows at the bottom.

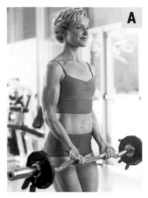
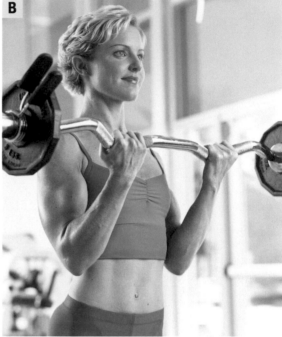

A B

The Next-Level Training Split

Day	Workout
1	Lower-Body Blast: medium effort
2	Upper-Body Blitz: medium effort
3	Rest
4	Lower-Body Blast: hard effort
5	Upper-Body Blitz: hard effort
6	Rest
7	Rest

Upper-Body Blitz

Exercise	WEEKS 1–2 Sets	WEEKS 1–2 Reps	WEEKS 3–4 Sets	WEEKS 3–4 Reps	WEEKS 5–6 Sets	WEEKS 5–6 Reps
CHEST						
Barbell Bench Press	3	10	3	8	3	6
Dumbbell Flye or Cable Crossover	3	12–15	3	12–15	3	12–15
BACK						
Lat Pulldown	3	10	3	8	3	6
Seated Cable Row	3	12–15	3	12–15	3	12–15
BICEPS						
EZ-Bar Curl	3	10	3	8	3	6
Machine Preacher Curl	3	12–15	3	12–15	3	12–15
TRICEPS						
Dumbbell Kickback	3	10*	3	8*	3	6*
Lying EZ-Bar Extension	3	12–15	3	12–15	3	12–15
SHOULDERS						
Dumbbell Upright Row	3	10	3	8	3	6
Seated Lateral Raise or Bent-Over Lateral Raise	3	12–15	3	12–15	3	12–15

* each side

Lower-Body Blast

Exercise	WEEKS 1–2 Sets	WEEKS 1–2 Reps	WEEKS 3–4 Sets	WEEKS 3–4 Reps	WEEKS 5–6 Sets	WEEKS 5–6 Reps
QUADRICEPS/GLUTES						
Front Squat	4	15	4	12	4	10
Stationary Barbell Lunge	4	15*	4	12*	4	10*
Single-Leg Squat	4	15*	4	12*	4	10*
HAMSTRINGS						
Romanian Deadlift	4	15	4	12	4	10
Lying Leg Curl	3	15	3	15	3	15
CALVES						
Calf Raise	3	15	3	15	3	15
Leg-Press Calf Raise	3	15	3	15	3	15
LOW BACK						
Back Extension	3	15	3	15	3	15
ABDOMINALS						
Crunch	3	15	3	15	3	15
Decline-Bench Crunch	3	15	3	15	3	15
Reverse Crunch	3	15	3	15	3	15
Exercise-Ball Crunch	3	15	3	15	3	15

*each side

Single-Leg Squat

Stand erect 3–4 feet in front of either an exercise ball (more challenging) or a flat bench placed behind you. Extend one leg back and place that foot on top of the bench/ball. With your hands on your hips or holding dumbbells, lower your hips by bending both knees until your front thigh is parallel to the floor. Don't allow your front knee to move past your toes. Focusing on your glutes, press back up through your front foot to the starting position and repeat for reps, then switch legs.

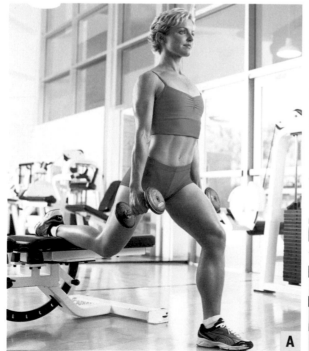
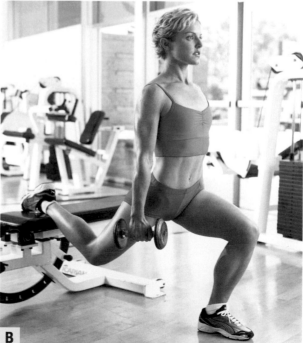

A B

GETTING STARTED | This whole-body work-out boosts intensity and calorie burn via supersets. Within each pair of exercises, rest only as long as it takes to set up your second exercise, and rest no longer than a minute between supersets.

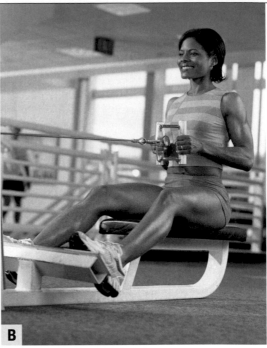

Seated Cable Row

Grasp the neutral V-grip handle and sit on the bench, feet flat on the platform. Keep your knees slightly bent, torso upright, abs tight and back slightly arched. Pull the handle toward your waist, keeping your arms close to your sides. Bring your elbows as far back as possible and squeeze your shoulder blades together. Slowly extend your arms to return to the start, keeping your back erect.

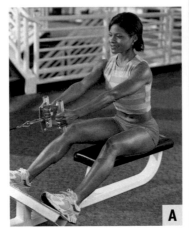

A B

The Super-Body Routine

Exercise	Sets	Reps
CHEST		
Incline Dumbbell Flye —superset with—	3	8
BACK		
Seated Cable Row	3	8
SHOULDERS		
Lateral Raise —superset with—	3	12
LOW BACK		
Back Extension	3	12
TRICEPS		
Straight-Bar Pressdown —superset with—	3	8
BICEPS		
Standing Cable Curl	3	8
QUADS		
Leg Extension —superset with—	3	8
HAMSTRINGS		
Lying Leg Curl	3	8
ABS		
Reverse Crunch —superset with—	3	8
CALVES		
Seated Calf Raise	3	8

Reverse Crunch

Lie faceup on the floor, bend your knees, lift your legs 90 degrees from your hips and place your hands under your low back. Contract through your lower abs to slowly curl your pelvis off the floor and toward your ribcage.

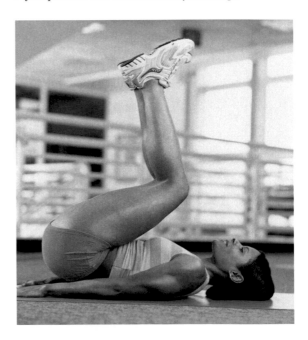

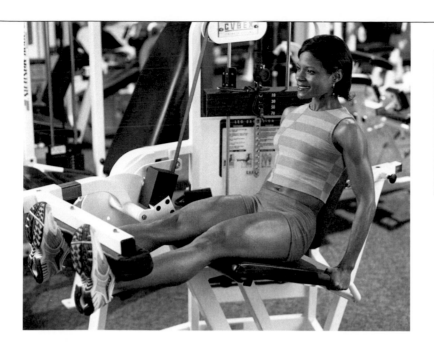

Leg Extension

Sit in the machine, adjusting the backpad so your knees are just beyond the edge of the seat and your back and thighs are flush against the pads. Push the ankle pad all the way up by extending your legs, squeeze your quads as hard as you can without locking your knees and return slowly, resisting the weight. Stop short of allowing the plates to rest on the stack to keep tension on the muscles.

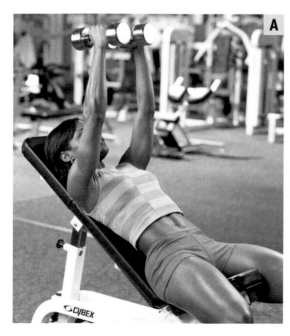

A B

Incline Dumbbell Flye

Lie faceup on a bench set to a 45-degree angle with your back and hips fully supported. Hold dumbbells directly over your shoulders, palms facing in and elbows slightly bent. Lower the weights out to your sides in an arc, stopping when your upper arms are parallel to the floor. Squeeze your chest to follow the same arc on the return.

>>tip

Working out at home?

INSTEAD OF:	DO:
Seated Cable Row	Bent-Over Dumbbell Row
Straight-Bar Pressdown	Bench Dip
Standing Cable Curl	Dumbbell Curl

Do back extensions off the floor or an exercise ball, and leg extensions and curls with a dumbbell held between your feet.

GETTING STARTED | In this total-body super-set workout, choose dumbbells that allow you to perform about 12 reps on the first exercise and as many reps as you can on the second. Move quickly, resting no more than a minute between exercise pairings.

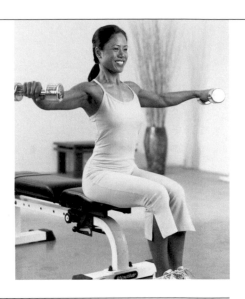

Seated Lateral Raise

Sit erect at the end of a flat bench or chair. Hold dumbbells alongside your hips with your palms facing in and your elbows bent slightly. Lift the weights up and out to shoulder level while keeping that slight bend in your elbows. For maximum contraction, your wrists, elbows and shoulders should be aligned at the top. Control the descent.

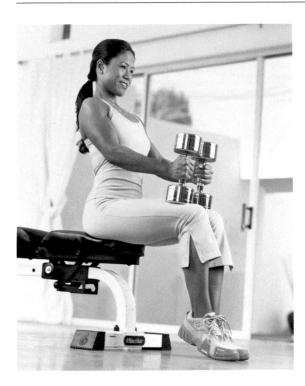

Dumbbell Calf Raise

Sit erect at the end of a flat bench, legs and feet together. Hold dumbbells so the flat ends rest just above your knees. Rise up onto your toes and squeeze your calves, then return to the floor.

At-Home Dumbbell Routine

Exercise	Sets	Reps
CHEST		
Dumbbell Flye	3	12
—superset with—		
Dumbbell Bench Press	3	12
SHOULDERS		
Seated Lateral Raise	3	12
—superset with—		
Seated Overhead Dumbbell Press	3	12
TRICEPS		
Lying Dumbbell Extension	3	12
—superset with—		
Seated Overhead Dumbbell Extension	3	12*
BACK		
Bent-Over Dumbbell Row	3	12
—superset with—		
Dumbbell Pullover	3	12
BICEPS		
Incline Dumbbell Curl	3	12
—superset with—		
Standing Dumbbell Curl	3	12
HAMSTRINGS & QUADS		
Walking Lunge	3	12*
—superset with—		
Back Squat	3	12
CALVES		
Dumbbell Calf Raise	3	15
—superset with—		
Calf Raise	3	15
ABS		
Reverse Crunch	3	15
—superset with—		
Crunch	3	15

*each side

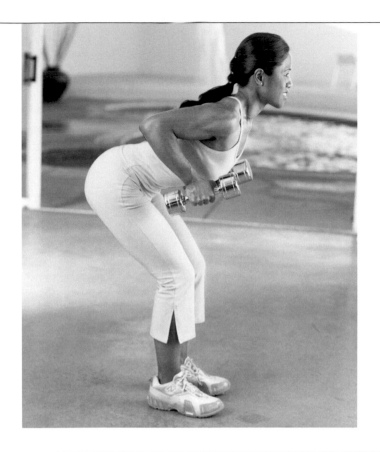

>>tip

The trick to burning more fat is to train all your major muscle groups, keeping the intensity high and your rest periods to a minimum. Beginners should do just one set per exercise.

Bent-Over Dumbbell Row

Lean forward with your feet about shoulder-width apart, knees slightly bent, a slight arch in your lower back. Start with the weights down in front of your legs, then squeeze your shoulder blades together and pull the weights up to your sides, keeping your elbows close to your body. Control the return.

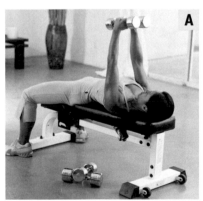

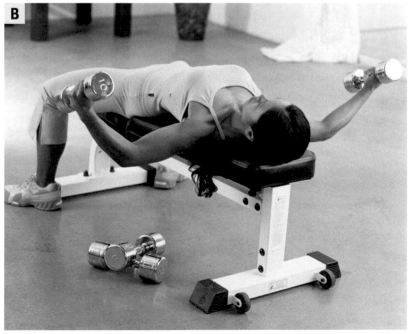

A B

Dumbbell Flye

Lie faceup on a flat bench holding dumbbells directly above your chest with your palms facing in. Slowly lower the weights straight out to your sides, keeping your elbows locked in a slight bend. Lower to arms-parallel, then squeeze your pecs to return to the start.

GETTING STARTED | Use this six-week inter-mediate program to boost your strength and cardiovascular base. Each workout builds on what you did the previous week. Using basic movements featured in this book, these routines advance your weight-training ability.

Week 1

Do circuit training plus cardio three times this week, allowing a day of rest between each full-body session. Don't worry about working at a particular exercise intensity or target heart rate yet, just keep moving! If the specified cardio equipment isn't available, use something else. Follow the program in order one time through.

Exercise	Reps
Brisk walk on treadmill	8 minutes
Exercise-Ball Squat	10
Push-Up	8–10
Standing Dumbbell Curl	8–10
Hands-Overhead Crunch	20
Stationary bike	8 minutes
Calf Raise (on step)	20
Lat Pulldown	8–10
Lateral Raise	8–10
Kick-Out	20
Elliptical climber	8 minutes
Stationary Lunge	8–10 each leg
Bench Dip	8–10
Straight-Leg Crunch	20

Reverse Decline Crunch

Lie faceup on a decline bench, grasping the rollers over your head. With your hips and knees bent 90 degrees, contract your abs to lift your glutes and bring your knees over your chest.

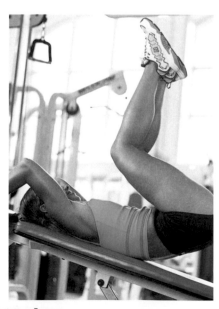

Week 2

This week, you'll do three full-body strength workouts with a day of rest between each. Rest 45–60 seconds between each set. Do all sets for an exercise before moving to the next. Do a cardio session on two of the days you don't lift weights.

Exercise	Sets	Reps
Back Squat	3	10
Lying Leg Curl	3	8
Barbell Bench Press	3	8–10
Lat Pulldown	3	8–10
Stationary Lunge (with 5–10-pound dumbbells)	3	10*
Calf Raise	3	15
Standing Overhead Dumbbell Press	3	10
Bench Dip^	3	6–10
EZ-Bar or Standing Dumbbell Curl	3	10
Reverse Decline Crunch	4	15

Cardio: Perform two sessions this week. Select three modes of cardiovascular exercise and work at 65% of your maximum heart rate for 10 minutes each. (To determine 65% of your maximum heart rate, subtract your age from 220 and then multiply that number by 0.65.) Options: treadmill hike at 10% incline, stationary bike, elliptical climber, rower, StepMill, stair-stepper, cross-country skiing machine. Cool down for 5–10 minutes at the end.

*each side ^Use two flat benches, placing your hands on the edge of one and your heels up on the other.

Week 3

This week, do three full-body strength workouts and three cardio sessions on separate days. Follow Week 2's program with the following modifications:

Back Squat: add 10–20 pounds
Barbell Bench Press: add 5–10 pounds
Lat Pulldown: add 1–3 more reps
Bench Dip: add 1–3 more reps
Reverse Decline Crunch: add five reps per set
Cardio: Add an extra cardio day from the previous week. Perform three cardio workouts and increase your time on each piece of equipment to 15 minutes, for a total of 45 minutes of cardio each day.

Week 4

Do three full-body workouts, two interval cardio sessions and enjoy two "fun fitness" days. Rest 90 seconds between the first two supersets; otherwise, rest 45–60 seconds.

Exercise	Sets	Reps
Plié Squat	3	10
—superset with—		
Lying Leg Curl	3	8
Incline Dumbbell Press	3	8–10
—superset with—		
One-Arm Dumbbell Row	3	8–10*
Reverse Lunge (with dumbbells)	3	20*
Standing Overhead Dumbbell Press	3	10
—superset with—		
Seated Alternating Dumbbell Curl	3	8
Adductor Machine	3	20
—superset with—		
Abductor Machine	3	20
(no rest between sets)		
Lateral Raise	3	10
—superset with—		
Dumbbell Kickback	3	10*
Seated Calf Raise^	3	20
Hanging Leg Raise	4	8–10
(rest long enough to catch your breath)		

Cardio: This week you'll start interval training, doing it twice a week on days you don't weight train. You can either walk, walk/run, jog/sprint or bike. Used by endurance athletes for improving speed and conditioning, intervals are fun and easy and can enhance your overall fitness level. First decide whether you're going to walk, run or bike, and whether you'll stay indoors or training outside. Then select a certain time frame; 20–30 minutes is usually enough. You may prefer to determine the length of the intervals by how you feel, rather than by time; you have lots of freedom to create your own workout.
Here's an example of interval training for a jog/run outside: Warm up with a light jog, then jog for 10 minutes. Pick a marker in the distance (stop sign, tree, lightpost, etc.) and run to that point. When you reach that point, jog until you feel recovered, then pick another marker to run to. Continue this alternating pattern of work/recovery for 20–30 minutes. Cool down with an easy jog and stretch. **On two other days,** select fun fitness activities.

*each side
^Mix it up every workout between standing, seated and donkey calf machine raises.

Week 5

This week you'll do three full-body strength workouts, two interval cardio sessions, one long cardio session and two "fun fitness" days. For all tri-sets and supersets, rest 60–90 seconds between each. For example, do one set each of the front squat, leg curl and stationary lunge, rest 60–90 seconds, then repeat two more times. Then move on to the push-up and lateral raise superset.

Exercise	Sets	Reps
Tri-Set:		
Front Squat	3	10
Lying Leg Curl	3	8
Walking Lunge	3	8*
Push-Up	3	10
—superset with—		
Lateral Raise	3	10
Wide-Grip Lat Pulldown	3	8–10
—superset with—		
Dumbbell Flye	3	10
Weighted Step-Up	3	10*
EZ-Bar Curl	3	10
—superset with—		
Front Dumbbell Raise	3	10
Adductor Machine	3	20
—superset with—		
Abductor Machine	3	20
(no rest between sets)		
Close-Grip Push-Up	3	8–10
—superset with—	3	10
Bent-Over Lateral Raise		
Ab Tri-Set:		
Bent-Knee V-Up	2	10
Bicycle	2	20
Crunch	2	30

Cardio: Do two interval workouts this week. Go harder than in previous workouts, running one minute, then recovering for no longer than 90 seconds. Keep the total workout time the same, but push a little more. For your one long cardio workout, select your favorite mode (running, swimming, elliptical climber, bike) or choose a few and split the time between them. Go long (60–75 minutes). On two other days, select fun fitness activities.

*each side

Week 6

Perform Week 5's program, but add a couple of reps on the push-ups and step-ups. Substitute the hanging knee raise to the side for the bent-knee v-up.

GETTING STARTED | At nearly every station in this circuit, you'll work for exactly 25 seconds. Since the time component is essential, either wear a watch with a second hand or have someone time you. Choose a weight that allows you to get just 12 reps in that 25 seconds.

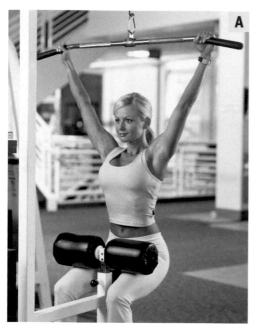

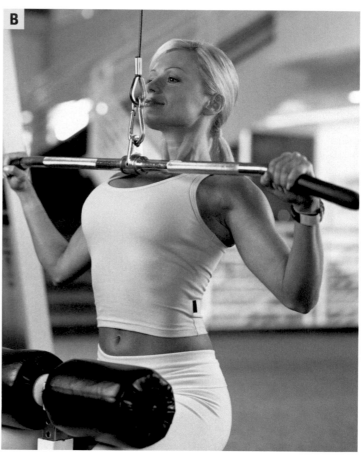

A | B

Lat Pulldown

Start by taking an overhand grip on the pulldown bar, slightly wider than shoulder width. Sit down and position your thighs under the pads, feet flat on the floor. Keep your back slightly arched and squeeze your shoulder blades together as you pull the bar down to your upper chest. Pause and return under control to the start position.

High-Power Circuit Routine

Exercise	CIRCUIT 1 Seconds/Reps*	CIRCUIT 2 Seconds/Reps*	CIRCUIT 3 Seconds/Reps*	CIRCUIT 4 Seconds/Reps*
Dumbbell Bench Press	25/12	25/12	25/11	25/10
Leg Press	25/12	25/12	25/11	25/10
Lat Pulldown	25/12	25/12	25/11	25/10
Crunch	25/15	25/15	25/15	25/0
Standing Overhead Dumbbell Press	25/12	25/12	25/11	25/10
Calf Raise	15/15	15/15	15/15	15/0
Lying Dumbbell Extension	25/12	25/12	25/11	25/10
EZ-Bar Preacher Curl	25/12	25/12	25/11	25/10
	Rest 30 sec.	Rest 30 sec.	Rest 30 sec.	

*Reps listed are a suggested goal; do as many as you can in 25 seconds. Go through the circuit as many times as it takes to complete the 45-rep goal.

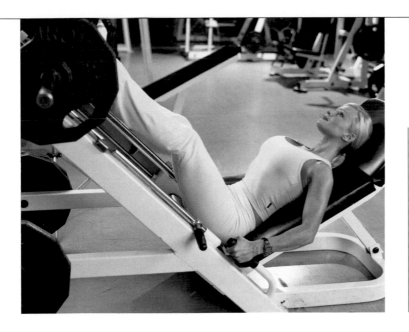

Leg Press

Sit in a leg-press machine, placing your feet high and slightly wider than shoulder-width apart on the platform. Keeping your back and hips flat against the pads, lower the sled until your knees form 90-degree angles. Pause briefly, then press back up to the starting position until your legs are straight but not locked. Focus on pressing through your heels for more glute emphasis. Don't lower the sled too far, which forces your lower back to lift off the backpad.

EZ-Bar Preacher Curl

Using an EZ-bar angles your wrists slightly and the bench stabilizes your arms when the pad supports most of your upper arms. Curl the weight up to where your elbows form roughly 90-degree angles, then lower it using a slow, controlled movement. Don't lock out; keep a slight bend in your elbows at the bottom. Make sure you lock your wrists to prevent flexing them as you bring the weight up, which would take some of the emphasis off the biceps.

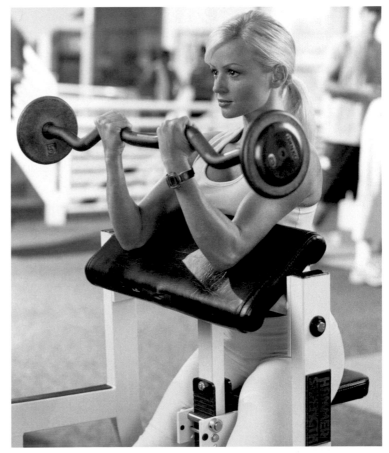

>>tip

When you reach the goal of 45 total reps of an exercise, eliminate it from the circuit. If you still have more reps of other movements to complete, rest for 25 seconds when you come to that station again. Try to complete the circuit in less than 30 minutes.

101

GETTING STARTED | A more traditional program with a twist, this alternates bouts of cardio with a 10-exercise circuit. Complete one set of 10–12 reps for each movement, using a weight that makes the last few reps very challenging. Move quickly between exercises.

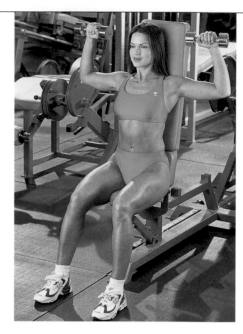

Seated Overhead Dumbbell Press

Sit erect on a bench with a back support, holding dumbbells at about ear level so your upper arms are roughly parallel to the floor, elbows close to 90 degrees. Press the dumbbells overhead, then lower under control.

Challenge Circuit Routine

Exercise	Reps
Machine Press	10–12
Pec-Deck or	10–12
Incline Dumbbell Flye	10–12
Lat Pulldown	10–12
Seated Overhead	10–12
Dumbbell Press	
Seated Lateral Raise	10–12
Horizontal Leg Press	10–12
Walking Lunge	10–12*
Seated Cable Row	10–12
Supinating Dumbbell Curl	10–12
Seated Overhead	10–12*
Dumbbell Extension	
8-minute Cardio Challenge	
REPEAT Circuit	
8-minute Cardio Challenge	
REPEAT Circuit	
5 Minutes Cool-Down + 3 Minutes Abs	
*each side	

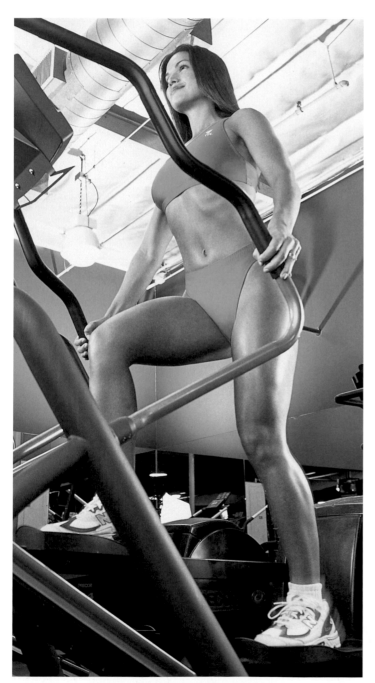

Cross-Body Crunch

Lie faceup on the floor, knees bent 90 degrees, and place one hand lightly behind your head. Curl up using the strength of your abs to lift your shoulder blade off the floor, then twist your torso to bring your shoulder as far as possible toward the opposite hip. Lower slowly, keeping your abs tight on the return. Alternate reps to each side.

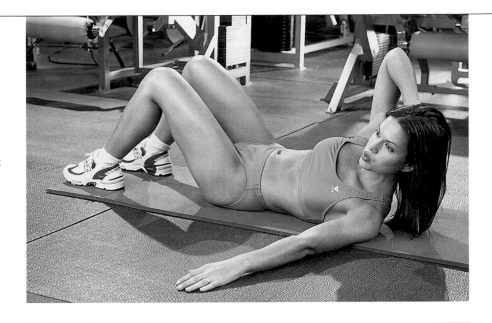

Supinating Dumbbell Curl

Stand erect with your elbows fixed at your sides, palms facing in. Contract your biceps to curl one weight at a time toward your shoulders, turning your wrist so your palm faces up at the top. Return along the same path without locking out your elbows at the bottom. You can also try holding one dumbbell in the top position while you curl the other.

>>tip

Challenge yourself during the eight-minute cardio intervals, doing the first four minutes at a moderate intensity, then upping your pace, incline and/or resistance for the last four minutes.

Index